The Pediatric Pes Planovalgus Deformity

Guest Editor

NEAL M. BLITZ, DPM, FACFAS

CLINICS IN PODIATRIC MEDICINE AND SURGERY

www.podiatric.theclinics.com

Consulting Editor
THOMAS ZGONIS, DPM, FACFAS

January 2010 • Volume 27 • Number 1

SAUNDERS an imprint of ELSEVIER, Inc.

W.B. SAUNDERS COMPANY
A Division of Elsevier Inc.

1600 John F. Kennedy Boulevard • Suite 1800 • Philadelphia, Pennsylvania 19103-2899

http://www.theclinics.com

CLINICS IN PODIATRIC MEDICINE AND SURGERY Volume 27, Number 1
January 2010 ISSN 0891-8422, ISBN-13: 978-1-4377-1863-8

Editor: Patrick Manley

Clinics in Podiatric Medicine and Surgery (ISSN 0891-8422) is published quarterly by Elsevier Inc., 360 Park Avenue South, New York, NY 10010-1710. Months of issue are January, April, July, and October. Business and Editorial Offices: 1600 John F. Kennedy Blvd., Ste. 1800, Philadelphia, PA 19103-2899. Customer Service Office: 3251 Riverport Lane, Maryland Heights, MO 63043. Periodicals postage paid at New York, NY and additional mailing offices. Subscription prices are $252.00 per year for US individuals, $367.00 per year for US institutions, $130.00 per year for US students and residents, $303.00 per year for Canadian individuals, $454.00 for Canadian institutions, $359.00 for international individuals, $454.00 per year for international institutions and $184.00 per year for Canadian and foreign students/residents. To receive student/resident rate, orders must be accompanied by name of affiliated institution, date of term, and the *signature* of program/residency coordinator on institution letterhead. Orders will be billed at individual rate until proof of status is received. Foreign air speed delivery is included in all *Clinics* subscription prices. All prices are subject to change without notice. POSTMASTER: Send address changes to *Clinics in Podiatric Medicine and Surgery*, Elsevier Health Sciences Division, Subscription Customer Service, 3251 Riverport Lane, Maryland Heights, MO 63043. **Customer Service: 1-800-654-2452 (US). From outside of the US, call 314-447-8871. Fax: 314-447-8029. E-mail: JournalsCustomerService-usa@elsevier.com (for print support); JournalsOnlineSupport-usa@ elsevier.com (for online support).**

Reprints. For copies of 100 or more of articles in this publication, please contact the Commercial Reprints Department, Elsevier Inc., 360 Park Avenue South, New York, NY 10010-1710. Tel.: 212-633-3812; Fax: 212-462-1935; E-mail: reprints@elsevier.com.

Clinics in Podiatric Medicine and Surgery is covered in *MEDLINE/PubMed (Index Medicus)* and *EMBASE/Excerpta Medica.*

Printed and bound in the United Kingdom
Transferred to Digital Print 2011

CLINICS IN PODIATRIC MEDICINE AND SURGERY

CONSULTING EDITOR
THOMAS ZGONIS, DPM, FACFAS

Contributors

CONSULTING EDITOR

THOMAS ZGONIS, DPM, FACFAS
Associate Professor and Chief, Division of Podiatric Medicine and Surgery, Department of Orthopaedic Surgery, University of Texas Health Science Center San Antonio, San Antonio, Texas; Director, Reconstructive Foot and Ankle Fellowship, University of Texas Health Science Center at San Antonio, San Antonio, Texas

GUEST EDITOR

NEAL M. BLITZ, DPM, FACFAS
Chief of Foot Surgery, Department of Orthopaedic Surgery, Bronx-Lebanon Hospital Center, Albert Einstein College of Medicine, Bronx, New York

AUTHORS

HOWARD BARKAN, DrPH
Joint Medical Program, School of Public Health, University of California, Berkeley, Berkeley, California

ANIL BHAVE, PT
Division Head, Rehabilitation; Director, Wasserman Gait Laboratory, Rubin Institute for Advanced Orthopedics, Sinai Hospital of Baltimore, Baltimore, Maryland

NEAL M. BLITZ, DPM, FACFAS
Chief of Foot Surgery, Department of Orthopaedic Surgery, Bronx-Lebanon Hospital Center, Albert Einstein College of Medicine, Bronx, New York

CLAIRE M. CAPOBIANCO, DPM
Fellow, Reconstructive Foot and Ankle Surgery and Clinical Instructor, Division of Podiatric Medicine and Surgery, Department of Orthopaedic Surgery, University of Texas Health Science Center at San Antonio, San Antonio, Texas

DANNY J. CHOUNG, DPM
Chief, Department of Podiatric Surgery, Kaiser Permanente, San Rafael, California

LAWRENCE A. DIDOMENICO, DPM
Adjunct Professor, Ohio College of Podiatric Medicine, Ohio; Director of Reconstructive Rearfoot and Ankle Surgical Fellowship; Chief, Section of Podiatric Medicine and Surgery, St Elizabeth Hospital, Youngstown, Ohio

MATTHEW B. DOBBS, MD
Associate Professor, Department of Orthopaedic Surgery, Washington University School of Medicine, St Louis, Missouri

SPYRIDON GALANAKOS, MD
Fourth Department of Orthopaedics, KAT General Hospital, Athens, Greece

RENATO J. GIORGINI, DPM
Section Chief Division of Podiatry, Good Samaritan Hospital Medical Center, West Islip, New York

MONIQUE C. GOURDINE-SHAW, DPM, LCDR, MSC, USN
Medical Service Corps, United States Navy, United States Naval Academy, Annapolis, Maryland; Veterans Affairs Maryland Healthcare Systems; Rubin Institute for Advanced Orthopedics, Sinai Hospital of Baltimore, Baltimore, Maryland

EDWIN J. HARRIS, DPM, FACFAS
Clinical Associate Professor of Orthopaedics and Rehabilitation, Section of Podiatry, Loyola University Medical Center, Maywood, Illinois

JOHN E. HERZENBERG, MD, FRCSC
Director, Pediatric Orthopedics; Director, International Center for Limb Lengthening, Rubin Institute for Advanced Orthopedics, Sinai Hospital of Baltimore, Baltimore, Maryland

BYRON HUTCHINSON, DPM, FACFAS
Highline Foot & Ankle Clinic, Franciscan Medical Group (part of Franciscan Health System), Seattle, Washington; Director of Podiatric Medical Education, Franciscan Foot & Ankle Institute, Saint Francis Hospital, Federal Way, Washington; Board of Directors, Northwest Podiatric Foundation, Edmonds, Washington

KLAUS J. KERNBACH, DPM
Attending Podiatric Surgeon and Research Director, Kaiser North Bay Consortium Residency Program, Department of Podiatry, Kaiser Foundation Hospital, Vallejo, California

BRADLEY M. LAMM, DPM, FACFAS
Head, Foot and Ankle Surgery, International Center for Limb Lengthening, Rubin Institute for Advanced Orthopedics, Sinai Hospital of Baltimore, Baltimore, Maryland

ANDREAS F. MAVROGENIS, MD
First Department of Orthopaedics, Attikon University of General Hospital, Athens University Medical School, Athens, Greece

JANAY MCKIE, MD
Department of Orthopaedic Surgery, The Mount Sinai Medical Center, New York, New York

PANAYIOTIS J. PAPAGELOPOULOS, MD, DSc
First Department of Orthopaedics, Attikon University of General Hospital, Athens University Medical School, Athens, Greece

TIMOTHY RADOMISLI, MD
Clinical Assistant Professor of Pediatric Orthopaedics, Department of Orthopaedic Surgery, The Mount Sinai Medical Center, New York, New York; Clinical Assistant Professor of Pediatric Orthopedics, Department of Orthopedic Surgery, Lenox Hill Hospital, New York, New York

CRYSTAL L. RAMANUJAM, DPM
Fellow, Postgraduate Research and Clinical Instructor, Division of Podiatric Medicine and Surgery, Department of Orthopaedic Surgery, University of Texas Health Science Center at San Antonio, San Antonio, Texas

NITZA RODRIGUEZ, DPM
Private Practitioner, Northern California Foot and Ankle Center, San Francisco, California

OLGA D. SAVVIDOU, MD
Department of Orthopaedics, Thriasio Hospital, Elefsina, Greece

ROBERT J. STABILE, DPM, AACFAS
Co-Chief, Division of Podiatry, Department of Surgery, Nassau University Medical Center, East Meadow, New York

RUSSELL G. VOLPE, DPM
Professor, Department of Orthopedics and Pediatrics, New York College of Podiatric Medicine, Foot Clinics of New York, New York, New York

THOMAS ZGONIS, DPM, FACFAS
Associate Professor and Chief, Division of Podiatric Medicine and Surgery, Department of Orthopaedic Surgery, University of Texas Health Science Center at San Antonio, San Antonio, Texas; Director, Reconstructive Foot and Ankle Fellowship, University of Texas Health Science Center at San Antonio, San Antonio, Texas

Contents

The frequent occurrence of flexible flatfoot raises the question of its pathologic status. There may be cultural overtones resulting in the consideration that flat feet are always pathologic. Parents may believe that their own flat feet were successfully treated when they were children and wish the same for their offspring. Few studies attempt to answer the question of the natural history of this condition. This article reviews the available literature dealing with the natural history, comorbidities, recommendations for treatment, expansion of biomechanical theory, and classification of flatfoot. Issues associated with imaging of flatfoot and the design of studies to validate the effects of treatment are also reviewed.

Many types of equinus exist in the pediatric population. This article reviews the causes, clinical and radiographic evaluation, and treatment of pediatric equinus deformity. It discusses the conservative and surgical management of the different types of equinus and when these treatments are best employed. The underlying pathophysiology for each equinus case must be understood to ensure that the treatment is appropriate.

The careful evaluation of the pediatric flatfoot begins with a detailed history and is followed by a thorough physical examination. Flatfeet may be congenital or acquired, and flexible or rigid. It is important to classify and evaluate a flatfoot, as the treatment recommendations depend on the assessment and proper diagnosis. The entire lower limb should be evaluated as a unit as one considers the suprapedal influences affecting foot position. The rigid flatfoot results in a fixed foot position that causes suprapedal compensation. On the other hand, most children presenting for evaluation of an acquired, flexible pes valgus deformity, with or without symptoms, will have abnormal, faulty biomechanical alignment of the lower extremity as the primary cause for an acquired, compensatory deformity of the foot

> Pediatric and adolescent flexible flatfoot is a pathomechanically complex deformity. Conservative and surgical treatment is directed at realigning the foot and alleviating symptoms. When surgical intervention is considered, there are various methods and techniques that may be performed to realign the foot. The treatment goals are directed first at resolution of pain, and second at the realignment of the foot. A specific treatment algorithm does not exist, although planal dominance influences direct the surgeons when considering surgical intervention. Open physis often dictates the direction of the reconstruction. Attempts at essential joint preservation should be strongly considered in this young patient population. This article provides an overview of the common treatment pathways that highlight methods to structurally realign the pediatric and adolescent flatfoot.

> Rigid pediatric pes planovalgus refers to a condition of the foot in which the medial longitudinal arch height is abnormally decreased along with a significant loss of midfoot and hindfoot motion in the pediatric patient. Known causes for this condition are well documented and consist of congenital vertical talus, tarsal coalitions, and peroneal spastic flatfoot without coalition. This article outlines conservative and surgical treatment of rigid pediatric pes planovalgus.

> Skewfoot is a rare condition that is often missed early in a child's development. Mild and flexible forms can be successfully treated with cast immobilization and shoe therapy. In more severe forms, surgical intervention is indicated if there are underlying neuromuscular conditions or the individual is affected on a daily basis because of the deformity. Careful evaluation and proper surgical procedures selection can realign the foot, resulting in favorable long-term outcomes. This article presents clinical and radiographic evaluation techniques and treatment options.

> Tarsal coalition is a congenital condition characterized by the aberrant union (osseous or fibrous) between 2 bones in the rearfoot, most commonly talocalcaneal coalition, calcaneonavicular coalition, and talonavicular coalition, that results in a restriction or absence of motion. The association between tarsal coalition and a variety of coexisting conditions has been reported over the past 60 years and continues to be better

understood. These coexisting conditions (the stigmata of tarsal coalition) have been believed to be secondary effects of the coalition and/or fixed rearfoot position. Advanced imaging has provided significant insights into the concomitant pathology and understanding of tarsal coalition that the symptoms associated with tarsal coalition can be present for a myriad of different reasons. One should consider all the stigmata of tarsal coalition when considering a surgical reconstruction.

Surgical reconstruction of symptomatic flatfoot associated with middle facet tarsal coalition is becoming more widely used. This article demonstrates that coalition-concomitant flatfoot is a pathologic entity that is worthy of surgical management. The literature, although limited, has suggested that poor outcomes with isolated simple coalition resection may have been related to the preoperative pes planus that was not addressed. More recently studies have demonstrated improved clinical and radiographic postoperative outcomes when the flatfoot correction is combined with the coalition resection. This article reviews a surgical treatment algorithm that considers the presence of varying degrees of pes planus and rearfoot arthrosis associated with coalition.

Symptomatic middle facet talocalcaneal coalition is frequently associated with rearfoot arthrosis that is often managed surgically with rearfoot fusion. However, no objective method for classifying the extent of subtalar joint arthrosis exists. No study has clearly identified the extent of posterior facet arthrosis present in a large cohort treated surgically for talocalcaneal coalition through preoperative computerized axial tomography. The authors conducted a retrospective review of 21 patients (35 feet) with coalition who were surgically treated over a 12-year period for coalition on at least 1 foot. Using a predefined original staging system, the extent of the arthrosis was categorized into normal or mild (Stage I), moderate (Stage II), and severe (Stage III) arthrosis. The association of stage and age is statistically significant. All of the feet with Stage III arthrosis had fibrous coalitions. No foot with osseous coalition had Stage III arthrosis. The distribution of arthrosis staging differs between fibrous and osseous coalitions. Only fibrous coalitions had the most advanced arthrosis (Stage III), whereas osseous coalitions did not. This suggests that osseous coalitions may have a protective effect in the prevention of severe degeneration of the subtalar joint. Concomitant subtalar joint arthrosis severity progresses with age; surgeons may want to consider earlier surgical intervention to prevent arthrosis progression in patients with symptomatic middle facet talocalcaneal coalition.

THE CLINICS ARE NOW AVAILABLE ONLINE!

Access your subscription at:
www.theclinics.com

Foreword
The Pediatric Pes Planovalgus Deformity

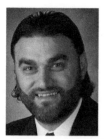

Thomas Zgonis, DPM, FACFAS
Consulting Editor

Congenital and acquired pediatric foot and ankle pathology poses a great challenge to surgeons. Knowledge of prenatal growth and foot development is paramount to understanding the pathophysiology of congenital deformities and how acquired deformities disrupt or alter this normal developmental pattern. Choosing the appropriate treatment depends on numerous variables unique to the pediatric population. Intervention through bracing, casting, or surgical reconstruction can have a profound impact on the growing foot. Certain deformities may be functionally less symptomatic as the patient matures, whereas other conditions and acquired deformities become more pronounced with severe functional limitations.

Dr Blitz and his colleagues have gathered detailed information on the most common pediatric conditions. This information will guide you in dealing with the pediatric lower extremity. Intervening on the growing foot is best understood and taught by those who have dedicated their entire practice or most of their practice to the pediatric population. For this dedication, I am thankful and applaud the guest editor and authors for their outstanding contributions and their dedication to this subspecialty of foot and ankle surgery.

Thomas Zgonis, DPM, FACFAS
Division of Podiatric Medicine and Surgery
Department of Orthopaedic Surgery
University of Texas Health Science Center San Antonio
7703 Floyd Curl Drive - MSC 7776
San Antonio, TX 78229, USA

E-mail address:
zgonis@uthscsa.edu

Clin Podiatr Med Surg 27 (2010) xv
doi:10.1016/j.cpm.2009.10.002
0891-8422/09/$ – see front matter

Preface
The Surgical Playbook

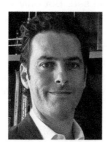

Neal M. Blitz, DPM, FACFAS
Guest Editor

Surgeons strive to gain control over the conditions with which they treat. There is a unique sense of clarity that occurs when one conquers a clinical problem. This feeling is intensified when there is harmony between one's hands, brain, and consciousness. Deep surgical understanding may be formulated over time or may occur as an epiphany.

Nonetheless, every surgeon develops an individualized "condition-based internal algorithm" that dictates how a particular problem should be managed. This "surgical playbook" is one's most valued asset as it is a compilation of the professional experience. It is a book like no other and cannot be bought, copied, or gifted to you. You must write all of its contents. It contains pages from your medical education, residency, fellowship, and working experience. It is the sum of your successes as well as your trials and tribulations.

The surgical playbook is referred to with every patient encounter and in every operative session. Conditions that are treated frequently are bookmarked and easily found. Those algorithms are "simple" and perfected. The ability to manage one condition does not necessarily guarantee that another more complex condition will be treated as flawlessly as conditions already dominated. There is an order to the book, and turning the page requires that one possesses the requisite skills and knowledge of the previous chapter.

Understanding and successfully managing pediatric and adolescent flatfoot is one of those conditions that is an advanced chapter in your book. Because flatfoot often has a variable presentation, its treatment plans are also variable. Patients may present with mild, moderate, or severe forms, as well as have multiplanar deformity. The flatfoot may be flexible or rigid, congenital or acquired, or occur with skeletal immaturity. Therefore, developing a surgical plan requires thoughtful decision-making and possession of a multivolume appended playbook without blank pages.

Clin Podiatr Med Surg 27 (2010) xvii–xviii
doi:10.1016/j.cpm.2009.10.001
0891-8422/09/$ – see front matter © 2010 Elsevier Inc. All rights reserved.

Remember that other surgeons have their own surgical playbook with treatment plans and algorithms that may be completely different to yours, yet achieve successful outcomes. This is often the case with flatfoot, in that there are multiple treatment pathways that may lead to the same desired outcome. Similar to a blivet, depending on how you interpret the image [condition] will determine what you see. But only with experience will you appreciate that conquering the impossible may not be as important as simply understanding it.

It should be clear that pediatric and adolescent flatfoot is complex, and there is no single page of your playbook that will provide you with every answer. The purpose of this issue of *Clinics* is to provide surgeons with an up-to-date resource on this continually evolving topic. Perhaps pages from this particular *Clinics* will find their way into your surgical playbook.

Neal M. Blitz, DPM, FACFAS
Chief of Foot Surgery
Department of Orthopaedic Surgery
Bronx-Lebanon Hospital Center
Albert Einstein College of Medicine
Bronx, NY

E-mail address: nealblitz@yahoo.com

The Natural History and Pathophysiology of Flexible Flatfoot

Edwin J. Harris, DPM, FACFAS

KEYWORDS

- Flatfoot • Flexible flatfoot • Physiologic flatfoot
- Nonphysiologic flatfoot • Planal dominance

Flat feet in infants, children, and adolescents are so common that the lack of agreement about the natural history and pathophysiology of the condition is surprising. There is great controversy about the role that flat feet play in health, and disagreement on the indications for treatment. The frequent occurrence raises the question of whether many of the mild forms are really a part of normal development and not a sign of disease.

Flat feet are considered by parents and some physicians as diseased, deformed, and in need of treatment simply because they exist. Staheli[1,2] suggested that part of this attitude may be cultural, because high arches have long been considered a sign of aristocracy, virtue, and well-being and therefore, good. Lower arches were traditionally considered a deformity, evidence of poor health, and something that needed to be treated and therefore bad.[1,2] It is the deviation from some ideal foot structure that supposedly makes flatfoot abnormal and presumably will result in long-term morbidity and disability in adulthood. Conversely, high-arched feet are indicators of muscle imbalance and are signs of underlying conditions that include static encephalopathy, myopathy, spinal dysraphisms, and other serious pathologic conditions. Triathletes with supinated foot types are more likely to sustain overuse injuries.[3] Manoli and Graham[4] regarded subtle cavoid feet as underpronators. This raises the question of whether most forms of flat feet constitute a morbid process with the characteristic symptoms and distinct natural history that, if left unmodified, will prove to be disabling. Only then does flatfoot meet the definition of a disease. Flatfoot becomes a medical issue only when symptoms develop. The mere absence of a well-formed medial longitudinal arch does not necessarily imply a pathologic condition.[5]

Flat feet continue to generate parental concern and result in many visits to health care professionals for consultation and treatment. Parents themselves may have been diagnosed with flat feet when they were children. They may have worn special

Department of Orthopaedics and Rehabilitation, Section of Podiatry, Loyola University Medical Center, Loyola University Chicago, Maguire Building Room 1700, 2160 South First Avenue, Maywood, IL 60153, USA
E-mail address: eharrisdpm@AOL.com

Clin Podiatr Med Surg 27 (2010) 1–23
doi:10.1016/j.cpm.2009.09.002
0891-8422/09/$ – see front matter

podiatric.theclinics.com

shoes, orthoses, or perhaps had surgery. They may be convinced that the treatments they received gave them a better prognosis and wish the same for their children. They may be aware of contributing factors that include genetics, ligamentous laxity, and association with other named syndromes. Their presumption is that available treatment influences the natural history of flatfoot in a positive way and brings about a long-term change in the function and the anatomy of the child's feet. If told by a physician that the child needs no treatment, parents may shop from doctor to doctor until they find someone who will satisfy their perceived needs.

There are huge gaps in our knowledge about flatfoot. Terminology of foot movement is confusing.[6,7] There is no agreement on a name for this entity. It is variously referred to as flatfoot, pes planus, pes valgoplanus, pes planovalgus, talipes valgus, and pronation syndrome. It is an anatomic lesion and not a diagnosis or even a single condition. It is a collection of clinical entities that are grouped together because they share similar features.

It is unfortunate that the term "flatfoot" enjoys such universal usage. It is misleading because it concentrates only on the sagittal plane component and the foot surface contact area, to the exclusion of the other planes. A literature review identified 22 articles dealing with height of the navicular from the floor and "navicular drop."[8–29] Flatfoot is a triplane deformity. Although the deformity is on 3 planes, 1 plane often dominates. Newer additions to biomechanical theory call this planal dominance.[30,31] As research continues, there is less concentration on the subtalar joint and more on the talocalcaneonavicular joint complex (the acetabulum pedis).[32–35]

The American College of Foot and Ankle Surgeons sponsored a project to develop clinical pathways for clinical diagnosis and treatment recommendations.[36] Published in 2004, the investigators identified several subsets of pediatric flatfoot, including flexible flatfoot, rigid flatfoot, skewfoot deformity, and flatfoot associated with some more specific diagnoses. Talipes calcaneovalgus and oblique talus deformity were not included in this classification, even though talipes calcaneovalgus is often referred to as "infantile flatfoot."[37–39]

Flexible flatfoot was divided into physiologic and nonphysiologic flatfoot. Nonphysiologic flatfoot may be asymptomatic or symptomatic. Rigid flatfoot was divided into congenital convex pes valgus, flatfoot associated with tarsal coalition, peroneal spastic flatfoot without tarsal coalition, and iatrogenic flatfoot. Skewfoot combines severe rearfoot pronation and rigid forefoot adductovarus. Flat feet associated with other issues are caused by neurologic disease, muscular disease, syndromes, and collagen vascular disease. There is no progressive relationship between flexible flatfoot and rigid deformities. Simple flatfoot does not become congenital convex pes valgus. Flexible flatfoot does not progress to rigid deformity in most cases.

There is difficulty even in defining flexible flatfoot. There is agreement that there is a normal arch when non–weight-bearing and a flattened arch when the child stands. It is hard to recognize the transition from the physiologic to the pathologic.[40–42] Nonphysiologic flexible flatfoot progresses over time instead of improving or at least stabilizing. It is more severe than physiologic flexible flatfoot and has excessive heel eversion with an unstable talonavicular joint. Tight heel cords and gait disturbance are commonly associated with nonphysiologic flatfoot. Children with equinus secondary to tight heel cords may benefit from stretching exercises, and, occasionally, heel cord lengthening. Orthoses may also be indicated.[43]

Most flexible flat feet are physiologic, asymptomatic, and require no treatment.[44–46] The natural history of physiologic flexible flatfoot is presumed to be one of improvement over time. Children with asymptomatic flexible flatfoot should be monitored clinically for development of symptoms and signs of progression. It is difficult to identify clinical factors in young children that may lead to a change in classification. Initial evaluation of the child should be thorough. Continued progression requires reassessment to search for underlying disease. Rigid flatfoot is identified by a stiff, flattened arch on and off weight-bearing. There is little argument that rigid flatfoot, skewfoot, and flatfoot associated with neuromuscular abnormalities, congenital syndromes, and collagen diseases are clearly pathologic and require treatment. There are no data available to suggest that these forms of flatfoot have any natural history that may result in clinical improvement over time. The status of flexible flatfoot is much less clear.

FLEXIBLE FLATFOOT

The controversy relates to that member of the flatfoot spectrum referred to as flexible flatfoot. Should all forms of flexible flatfoot be grouped together? Are all forms pathologic? There is little argument about the need to treat those forms of flatfoot that are clearly pathologic. There is a presumption that all flexible flatfoot is disease. Aggressive long-term management of all pronation has been advocated historically.[47] There is little discussion about the morbidity experienced by the child. It seems that it is the anatomic lesion that is considered to be objectionable. This leads to the question: if flexible flatfoot is a common issue, asymptomatic and without long-term morbidity, then when is treatment justified?

Asymptomatic flexible flatfoot is an almost universal finding in toddlers. This high frequency has been attributed to several things. One explanation is that the thickness of the plantar soft tissue is made up of "baby fat." This produces a plantigrade foot that may only appear flat. It is difficult to determine true flatness by physical examination alone. The only way is through evaluation of standardized weight-bearing antero-posterior (AP) and lateral radiographs of the feet. These can be difficult to obtain in small children, and radiographic techniques vary from investigator to investigator. Interpretation is complicated by incomplete ossification of the foot structures. The presumption that the ossific nuclei represent the true shape of the cartilaginous anlagen has been successfully challenged.[48–52] This makes radiologic interpretation difficult because age changes the location and shape of ossification centers until they become truly representative of the bone near skeletal maturity.

Other orthopedic variables also operate in this age group. Tibia varum is physiologic up to 2 years of age. Because this produces a varus or inverted tibial relationship to the support surface, the only way that the infant's medial column of the foot can reach the ground is for the rearfoot to pronate. By 2 years of age, most children have parallel tibias or genu valgum. At this time, the presence or absence of abnormal pronation becomes more evident. Toddlers have an abducted externally rotated gait pattern. This gait places the long axis of the foot external to the line of progression and allows propulsion off the medial side of the foot. There is also the mistaken notion that all abduction of the foot is a sign of pronation. In reality, abduction is likely to be supra-malleolar (**Fig. 1**).[44]

To summarize: factors that can modify the natural history of pediatric flexible flatfoot include ligamentous laxity, obesity, proximal rotational abnormalities, tibial influence, pathologic tibia varum, equinus, presence of an os tibiale externum, and presence of tarsal coalition.[53]

THE NATURAL HISTORY OF FLEXIBLE FLATFOOT

There are few studies on the natural history of flexible flatfoot if left untreated and on the subsequent natural history of the condition when it is treated. The available

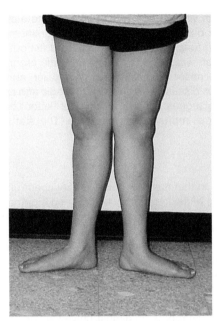

Fig. 1. A 12-year-old girl has severe external rotation of the lower extremities secondary to external tibial torsion and externally rotated hips. Although there is obvious pronated foot structure, the supramalleolar component produces the greatest component of the abducted gait.

literature is of questionable merit in the light of today's insistence on evidence-based medicine, levels of clinical evidence, and study construction. There are no data to conclusively prove that flexible flatfoot in infants and children leads to long-term morbidity in adults. The lack of agreement on the need to treat flexible flatfoot has resulted in the development of 2 polarized, dogmatic, and opposite philosophies regarding treatment. Today's physicians are forced to make decisions based on their personal training and experience and on conclusions drawn from the literature. It is difficult to evaluate the validity of these so-called authoritative conclusions. Some decisions are based on data, but many are "expert opinion." Even those based on data arrive at conclusions supported by statistical analyses that seem counterintuitive to common clinical experience.

This lack of data affects the evaluation of long-term benefits from the use of exercises, physical therapy, special shoes, and orthoses. One study dealing with the question of shoes and orthoses as modifiers of the natural history of flexible flatfoot shows how difficult it is to construct a valid scientific prospective study.[54] Interested readers should study the article by Wenger and colleagues[54] and the Editorial and the 2 Letters to the Editor that appeared in the same issue. Operative therapy is not immune to criticism and generates its own share of controversy. Surgical intervention certainly changes the anatomy, but it is permanent and not without risk. When potential morbidity and cost are factored in, it becomes even more imperative to demonstrate that such intervention is medically necessary and that therapy is likely to achieve the proposed goals.

There is a natural history to the development of the child's arch that cannot be denied. Staheli and colleagues[55] studied 441 normal subjects from 1 to 80 years of age and concluded that flat feet are usual in infants, common in children, and within the normal range of observations made in adult feet. Their recommendation for management was documentation and observation.

Gould and colleagues[56] studied 225 beginning walkers and followed them for 4 years. All of the apparently normal toddlers had pes planus determined by radiographic and photographic parameters. Arches developed regardless of the footwear worn. Children who had arch-support footwear developed arches faster. Hyperpronation was evident in 77.9% and genu valgum in 92.3% of the 5-year-olds.

Garcia-Rodriguez and colleagues[57] studied the prevalence of flexible flatfoot in a population of 4- to 13-year-old schoolchildren in Malaga, Spain. They graded by severity a sample of 1181 children from a total population of 198,858 primary school children. They made 3 age groups (4–5, 8–9, and 12–13 years old) and classified their footprints into 3 grades of flat feet. They found the prevalence of flat feet to be 2.7% of the 1181 children sampled. Of the patient sample, 168 (14.2%) were receiving orthopedic treatment, but only 2.7% met the diagnostic criteria for flat feet. Of the group that met the criteria for flat feet, only 28.1% were being treated. Overweight children in the 4- to 5-year-old age group had increased prevalence for flat feet. Their data suggested that an excessive number of children within the study group were being treated.

Lin and colleagues[58] studied flexible flatfoot in preschool children in Taiwan using gait analysis. Two hundred and seventy-seven preschool children (201 boys and 176 girls), from 2 to 6 years of age, were enrolled in the study. The results showed that age, height, weight, foot progression angle, occurrence of physiologic knock knees, and joint laxity scores correlated with flat feet. Children with flat feet, compared with children without, performed physical tasks poorly and walked slowly, as determined by gait parameters. They concluded that flatfoot should not simply be regarded as a problem of static alignment of the ankle and foot complex but may be a consequence of dynamic functional change in the whole lower extremity.

El and colleagues[59] studied longitudinal arch morphology in 579 schoolchildren and evaluated generalized joint laxity, foot progression angle, frontal-hindfoot alignment, and longitudinal arch. They evaluated 82.8% as normal and mild flatfoot, and 17.2% were evaluated as moderate and severe flexible flatfoot. There was a significant negative correlation between arch index and age and between hypermobility score and age.

Pfeiffer and colleagues[60] studied 835 children between the ages of 3 and 6 years, basing their diagnosis of flatfoot on a valgus position of the heel and poor formation of the arch. Prevalence of flexible flatfoot in the 3- to 6-year-old age group was 44%. Incidence of pathologic flatfoot was less than 1%. Ten percent of the children were wearing arch supports. The prevalence of flatfoot decreased by age from 54% in the 3-year-old age group to 24% in the 6-year-old age group. There were more boys than girls with flat feet (52% vs 36%). Obesity was a complication in 13%. They concluded that likelihood of flatfoot was influenced by age, gender, and weight. They concluded that more than 90% of the treatments instituted in their patient population were unnecessary.

Other investigators have studied specific populations to determine the relevance of flatfoot in adults and carry this information over to the pediatric population. The classic article by Harris and Beath[43] from 1948 not only described hypermobile flatfoot with short tendo-Achilles but also discussed some data from the 1944 to 1945 Royal Canadian Army Medical Corps study on Army foot problems. Among 3619 Canadian soldiers, there were 25 cases of severe hypermobile flatfoot with short tendo-Achilles, 192 cases of mild hypermobile flatfoot with short tendo-Achilles, 74 cases of peroneal spastic flatfoot, and 524 cases characterized by low arch. They further concluded that the natural history of hypermobile flatfoot with short tendo-Achilles is for it to become more severe, and more incapacitating, with increasing age. The disability is mild in childhood and may not be expressed until adolescence. It worsens in young adult life, and by middle life it may have reached severe proportions.[43]

Forriol and Pascual[61] studied the footprints of 1676 schoolchildren (1013 girls and 663 boys) between the ages of 3 and 17 years. They noted a high percentage of lowered medial longitudinal arches in the young age groups and a lower percentage in the older age groups. Their conclusion was that the medial longitudinal arch is a physiologic development in the earlier years of growth.

Cowan and colleagues[62] studied 246 US Army infantry trainees and their conclusions did not support the hypothesis that low-arched individuals are at increased risk of injury.

Rudzki[63] studied 350 men in the Australian Army and concluded that pes planus was not a significant factor in the development of injury during recruit training.

Hogan and Staheli[13] investigated the concept that treatment of flexible flatfoot in children will prevent disability in adult life. Proponents of not treating flexible flatfoot cite military studies that show that flexible flat feet are not a source of disability in soldiers. They studied 91 physically active civilian adult men and women and found no relationship between arch configuration and pain, suggesting that in the civilian population flexible flat feet are not a source of disability. They concluded that their study was consistent with previous studies and that it provided additional evidence against the practice of treating flexible flat feet in children.

Abdel-Fattah and colleagues[64] studied 2100 military recruits between the ages of 18 and 21 years in the Saudi Arabian Army. The incidence of flatfoot was 5%. Their conclusion was that family history, wearing shoes during childhood, obesity, and urban residency were significant issues associated with flatfoot. Because no flatfoot-related complaints were reported among the cases, their conclusion was that flexible flatfoot did not seem to be the cause of any disability.

DATA FROM FORMS OF IMAGING
Footprint Analysis

To diagnose and follow the natural history of flexible flatfoot, some sort of imaging must be used. Footprint recordings are inexpensive and easy to obtain, but more difficult to standardize and interpret. In addition, they merely represent the contact area of the plantar surface of the foot without giving any information on bony interrelationships. Radiographs are more frequently used but suffer the same problem with standardized positioning and angle-drawing techniques. Footprint and radiographic interpretations have issues with interobserver and intraobserver reliability.

El and colleagues[59] studied 579 primary school children and evaluated generalized joint laxity, foot progression angle, frontal-hindfoot alignment, and longitudinal arch height in dynamic positions. They used footprints obtained from the Harris-Beath mat and concluded that there is a negative correlation between arch height and age and between hypermobility score and age and that flexible flatfoot and hypermobility are developmental profiles.

Garcia-Rodriguez and colleagues[57] studied the incidence of flexible flatfoot in a population of 4- to 13-year-old schoolchildren and grouped their footprints into 3 flatfoot grades. They determined that the prevalence of flat feet was 2.7% of the 1181 children sampled.

Kanatli and colleagues[65] studied the relationship of radiologically measured angles and the arch index obtained from footprint analysis of 38 children with flexible flatfoot. They concluded that footprint analysis could be used effectively for screening studies and in individual office examinations.

Mickle and colleagues[66] used plantar footprints to study Australian preschool children to determine whether flatfoot was influenced by gender. They concluded that more boys had flat feet than girls. This finding was due to a thicker plantar fat pad in boys.

Radiology Analysis

Radiology has a historical role in the diagnosis and management of flat feet. Some studies relied heavily on this form of imaging. In the 1944 to 1945 Royal Canadian Army Medical Corps survey, all 3619 subjects had radiographs.[43]

Akcali and colleagues[8] studied 20 children with flexible flatfoot and external tibial torsion and a control group of 10 children with flexible flatfoot without rotational problems. Talar declination angle, talo–first metatarsal angle, and dorsoplantar talocalcaneal angles were measured on standing radiographs. Tibial torsion was measured by computed tomography (CT). They identified increased plantar talar declination and increased AP talocalcaneal angle. There was also prominent naviculocuneiform sag. Their conclusion was that abnormal external tibial torsion may affect the foot deformity and can change the benign nature of flexible flatfoot.

Harty[67] identified imaging pediatric foot disorders as a challenging task. He concluded that optimally exposed and well-positioned radiographs can answer many questions. CT and magnetic resonance imaging (MRI) are often needed to provide additional information to assist in the management of congenital and acquired foot lesions.[67] Positioning infants and young children can be difficult because of poor patient cooperation. Unless present during the exposure, the interpreter of the study is at the mercy of the technician.

Pehlivan and colleagues[68] evaluated the value of radiology to distinguish symptomatic and asymptomatic flexible flatfoot in young men. They concluded that an increased lateral talo–first metatarsal angle might be an important risk factor for development of symptoms in otherwise normal flexible flat feet.

Kuhn and colleagues[69] radiographically evaluated flexible pes planus patients with and without orthoses and concluded that there were statistically significant improvements in weight-bearing foot alignment with orthosis use. They concluded that their study supports the use of custom flexible orthotics for the improvement of pedal structural alignments.

Vanderwilde and colleagues[70] performed a radiographic measurement study of the feet in normal infants and children to establish standard radiographic values by evaluating weight-bearing radiographs of 74 normal infants and children admitted to a hospital for issues other than orthopedic disease. They ranged in age from 6 to 127 months and were grouped into 10 age groups. They examined AP, true lateral, and maximum dorsiflexion lateral radiographs. On the AP, the knees were flexed with the central ray directed at the talus. They measured the talocalcaneal angle, the calcaneus–fifth metatarsal angle, and the talus–first metatarsal angle. On the lateral radiograph, they measured the talocalcaneal angle, tibiocalcaneal angle, tibiotalar angle, talus–first metatarsal angle, and talo-horizontal angles. They also measured the talocalcaneal and tibiocalcaneal angles on stress dorsiflexion radiographs. The talocalcaneal index is calculated by adding the values of the AP and lateral talocalcaneal angles. Their results were that girls and boys and right and left feet had similar findings. AP talocalcaneal and fifth metatarsal–calcaneus angles decreased with age. Lateral talocalcaneal and talo–first metatarsal angles decreased less with age. Lateral tibiotalar, talo-horizontal, and maximum dorsiflexion talocalcaneal angles showed the least decrease with age.

Bleck and Berzins[71] studied flatfoot in children using the Helfet heel seats or the University of California Biomechanics Laboratory (UCBL) orthoses. They called this deformity pes valgus with plantarflexed talus, flexible. Follow-up examination of 71 cases revealed that 79% of the patients treated for more than a year had clinical and roentgenographic improvement. They recommended the Helfet heel seat if the plantarflexion angle of the talus is 35° to 45° and the UCBL shoe insert if plantarflexion of the talus is greater than 45°.

LEVELS OF EVIDENCE
Case-control Studies, Case Series, and Articles Primarily Expressing Expert Opinion

Based on levels of evidence for primary research, case-control studies (level III), case series (level IV), and articles relating primarily expert opinions (level V) are the least reliable. However, there are many such articles in the literature.

Bahler[44] discussed management of the more pronounced form of flexible flatfoot with the use of various types of insoles and also differentiated 5 components in the development of flexible flat feet. He concluded that a slight form of flatfoot is physiologic in children and that more pronounced forms require treatment.

Wenger and Leach[72] stated that flexible flatfoot is a manifestation of a constitutional laxity of ligaments and joints and seems abnormal because of weight-bearing stresses. They concluded that most children with flatfoot achieve a partial correction spontaneously and that current research at the time of their writing did not document that treatment with corrective shoes or inserts produced a result better than the partial correction that occurs naturally.

Jani[40] identified the difficulty in recognizing the transition of flexible flatfoot from a physiologic condition to a pathologic condition that makes assessment of therapy difficult. He questioned the usefulness of arch supports. However, he felt that the therapy was indicated for severe flatfoot deformities recognized by heel valgus of more than 20° and lack of a medial arch. Results of follow-up examinations of treated and untreated cases of flexible flat feet suggest that the value of the arch support insoles that are used widely is more than questionable.[40]

Zollinger and Fellmann[41] also noted the difficulty in separating normal variations of children's feet from pathologic conditions. It was their contention that flexible flatfoot disappears during growth. There was little pathologic significance if it persisted in adults. Differentiation is made between a benign pain-free course of development with no functional restrictions and pathologic deformities that require conservative or surgical therapy. Zollinger and Exner[42] stated that the spectrum of normal variations of children's feet is extremely broad and often difficult to separate from pathologic conditions. They concluded that flexible flatfoot normally disappears during growth. Even if it persists into adult life, it has no real pathologic significance. The natural course, even of severe flexible flatfoot in children, leads to good results that are often better than the surgical results, and more discretion with surgical treatment was advocated.

Cappello and Song[45] stated that infants are born with flexible flatfoot and that a normal arch develops in the first decade of life. They concluded that flexible flatfoot rarely causes disability, and asymptomatic children should not be burdened with orthotics or corrective shoes. Flexible flatfoot with tight heel cords may become symptomatic and can be addressed with a stretching program. Surgical intervention for flexible flatfoot is reserved for patients who have persistent localized symptoms despite conservative care. Rigid or pathologic flat feet have multiple causes, and many will require treatment to alleviate symptoms or improve function.

Hefti and Brunner[73] noted that many parents have anxiety about insufficient foot arches of their children. They stated that the arch is physiologically flattened by a hypervalgus of the hindfoot, and these feet do not need treatment.

Li and Leong[74] grouped intoeing gait, flexible flatfoot, bow legs, and knock knees in 1 category of physiologic problems that occur in normal children.

Sullivan[46] noted that the exact incidence of flatfoot in children is unknown but that it is a common finding. He further stated that all children have only a minimal arch at birth, and more than 30% of neonates have calcaneovalgus deformity of both feet. He concluded that calcaneovalgus is not painful and generally resolves without treatment. The same thing is true of flexible flatfoot. His recommendation was that the examining physician must rule out the existence of those conditions that do require treatment.

Attempts at Higher Level Studies

Whitford and Esterman[29] performed a randomized controlled trial of 2 types of in-shoe orthoses in children with flexible excessive pronation of the feet between the ages of 7 and 11 years. They made the diagnosis by observing calcaneal eversion and navicular drop. They found no evidence to justify the use of in-shoe orthoses in the management of flexible excessive pronation in children.

Evans studied the relationship between "growing pains" and foot posture in children, investigating the complaint of aching legs and its relation to pronated foot posture using 8 single-case experimental designs. The foot posture is believed to be deleterious and is often treated with in-shoe devices. This intervention proved helpful for children with pronated foot posture and aching legs.[75] Four years later, Evans and Scutter[76] compared foot posture with functional health between children aged 4 to 6 years with and without leg pain and reached the conclusion that navicular height was not predictive for growing pains. They also concluded that there was no support for the anatomic theory for growing pains and did not find a meaningful relationship between foot posture or functional health measures and leg pain in young children.[76]

PATHOPHYSIOLOGY

Understanding of the pathology of flatfoot is based on anatomic experimental data, theoretical biomechanics, and clinical observations in patient care. Anatomic studies dating back to the 1930s and 1940s led to the Root biomechanical theory of foot function. This approach to foot abnormality relies heavily on subtalar joint biomechanics and coronal plane forefoot-to-rearfoot interrelationship. As a natural consequence of gaining knowledge, the Root approach to foot biomechanics is not so much being challenged as being added to.

Much of Root biomechanical theory is based on the subtalar joint neutral position. However, it is impossible to anatomically define the subtalar joint neutral position with any degree of precision. At least 4 techniques have been described. First, it is traditionally defined as the position the calcaneus occupies when it is placed at one-third of the total subtalar range of motion moving from the position of full eversion. A second technique involves lining up the lateral calcaneus with the fibula. A third technique is palpating for full coverage of the talar head by the navicular. Fourth, it has been described as that position in which the foot is neither pronated nor supinated.

Kirby[77] introduced the concept of foot function based on the spatial location of the subtalar joint axis in relation to the weight-bearing structures in the plantar foot, using the concept of subtalar joint rotational equilibrium to explain how externally generated forces, such as ground reaction forces, and internally generated forces, such as ligamentous and tendon tensile forces, and joint compression forces affect the mechanical behavior of the foot and lower extremity.

McPoil and Cornwall[78] found that, contrary to previously published theory, the "neutral" position of the rearfoot for the typical pattern of rearfoot motion during the walking cycle was found to be the resting rather than subtalar joint neutral position. It is clear that equating flatfoot pathology with subtalar joint function is a gross oversimplification of an extremely complicated anatomic area.

Ball and Afheldt[79] challenged the Root orthotic theory and stated that the casting and evaluation techniques have poor reliability and unproven validity and that the principles are rarely followed. They also challenged the concept that excessive foot eversion leads to excessive pronation and that orthotics provided beneficial effects by controlling rearfoot inversion and eversion. It was their contention that control of internal/external tibial rotation is the most significant factor in maintaining proper supination and pronation mechanics. They also suggested that proprioceptive influences play a large role.

Detailed discussion of the pathophysiology of flexible flatfoot is outside of the scope of this article. However, the highlights can be stressed. Too much of the literature concentrates on abnormal foot-to-surface contact and failure of foot structure on the sagittal plane (loss of the medial arch). Abnormal pronation is triplanar. It is usual to find deformity on all 3 planes, but it is more pronounced on 1 plane. This tendency has led to the concept of planal dominance.[30] By recognizing the plane of the greatest component of the deformity, treatment options can be more accurately selected. Coronal (frontal) plane deformity is recognized by marked increase in subtalar eversion motion. Transverse plane pronation is recognized by transverse talonavicular instability without excessive heel eversion and without failure of the medial column in the sagittal plane. Sagittal plane pronation can be identified by breech along the medial column. This condition can be seen on clinical inspection but is more apparent on weight-bearing lateral radiographs. More emphasis is currently being placed on evaluating the rearfoot as if it were a complex functional talocalcaneonavicular joint unit (the acetabulum pedis).[32–35]

There are certain aspects of the pathophysiology of flatfoot that are not controversial. Painful pronated foot structures with rearfoot rigidity are often caused by tarsal coalitions. Barroso and colleagues[80] placed the incidence of congenital tarsal coalition at about 1% and recognized it as the main cause of painful rigid flatfoot in the pediatric population. Blakemore and colleagues[81] also identified tarsal coalitions as a major cause of painful rigid flat feet in children and adolescents. They identified the most common types as talocalcaneal and calcaneonavicular coalitions. Lowy[82] discussed pediatric peroneal spastic flatfoot in the absence of coalition.

The cause of flexible flatfoot is unknown. There is evidence that there are genetic tendencies toward excessive pronation. It is not unusual to see flexible flatfoot in multiple siblings and to trace it back through several generations. Additional diagnoses, such as ligamentous laxity and hypotonia, are often combined with flexible flatfoot. This combination is often the point at which flexible flatfoot ceases to be physiologic and becomes pathologic.

Flexible flatfoot can be influenced by tibia varum, genu valgum, gastrosoleus contracture, and primary ankle joint valgus. Primary ankle joint valgus is often overlooked in the assessment of pronated feet. If it is present, foot eversion becomes the sum of subtalar eversion plus supramalleolar valgus (**Fig. 2**). Obesity also adversely modifies the course of flexible flatfoot and may be a major cause for foot and leg discomfort.

Planal Dominance

From the pathophysiologic point of view, flexible flatfoot is identified by abnormal subtalar joint pronation, some degree of transverse plane uncovering of the talonavicular joint, and flatness of the medial longitudinal arch. There are 4 types of flexible flatfoot based on the concept of planal dominance. The first is coronal or frontal plane pronation, characterized by abnormal eversion of the calcaneus in the coronal plane. It is difficult to attach specific numbers to calcaneal eversion, but more than 15° is considered excessive (**Fig. 3**).

Transverse plane pronation is characterized by uncovering of the talar head medially at the talonavicular joint in the absence of excessive heel eversion. This condition increases the AP talocalcaneal angle and results in some degree of abduction of the lateral forefoot. Calcaneal eversion rarely exceeds 10°. Lateral radiographs are surprisingly normal. There is little or no failure of the medial column in the sagittal plane. It gives the impression that the lateral column is short (**Fig. 4**).

Sagittal plane pronation involves the other 2 planes, but the defining feature is failure of the medial column at the talonavicular joint, the cuneonavicular joint, the first metatarsocuneiform joint, or at several of these locations (**Fig. 5**).

Triplane pronation shows excessive heel eversion, transverse plane talar head uncovering, and collapse of the medial column without any real dominance on any of the planes (**Fig. 6**).

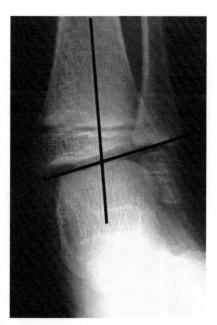

Fig. 2. In the workup for pronated feet, the possibility that the ankle joint may not be horizontal must be taken into consideration. If there is primary ankle valgus deformity, the calcaneus is everted with reference to the weight-bearing surface independent of any subtalar joint position. This condition cannot be modified by any in-shoe orthosis.

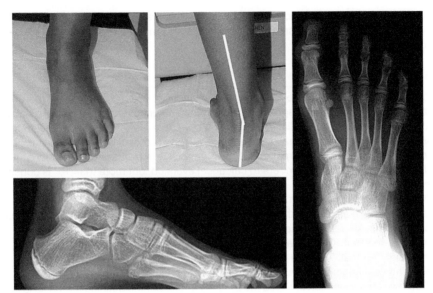

Fig. 3. Coronal plane dominant pronation without change on the remaining planes. There is marked heel eversion noted clinically. The radiographs show a normal AP talocalcaneal angle and normal lateral talocalcaneal relationship with preservation of the medial column.

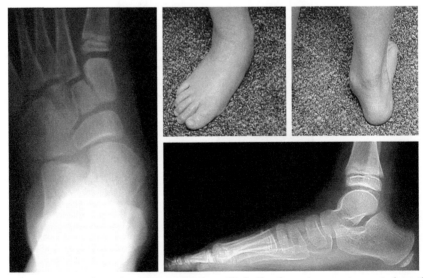

Fig. 4. Transverse plane dominant pronation. Clinically, the calcaneus is everted to the weight-bearing plane and the forefoot is abducted on the rearfoot. The radiographs show much of the medial talar head uncovered on the AP radiograph, with minimal failure of the medial column in the sagittal plane on the lateral radiograph.

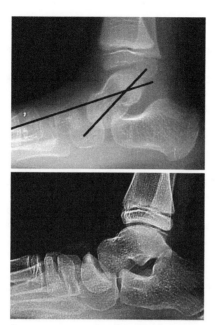

Fig. 5. Sagittal plane dominant pronation. Medial column collapse may be at the talonavic-ular joint or at some point distal.

Forefoot varus is often a manifestation of sagittal plane dominant deformity. In pediatric practice, the incidence of forefoot varus before the age of 6 years is almost nonexistent, which suggests that much of the adult forefoot varus is acquired.

The importance of equinus deformity as a complication of pronation cannot be overemphasized. Like forefoot varus, congenital equinus in the pediatric age group is uncommon. If present, the congenital form is almost always associated with neuromuscular disease. Acquired equinus is first seen toward the end of the first decade

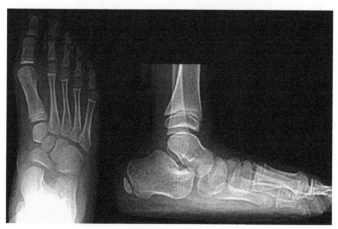

Fig. 6. Triplane pronation. The AP and lateral radiographs show equal signs of pronation. The transverse and sagittal planes are affected.

of life. If there is inadequate ankle joint dorsiflexion, the lack of ankle movement has to be compensated for by pronating the rearfoot, or the heel cannot reach the ground. This method may require maximal or supramaximal pronation to the point at which joint surfaces are actually subluxed (**Fig. 7**).

The angle made by the tibia and the weight-bearing plane is also important. In children younger than 2 years, physiologic tibia varum is seen. To get the medial forefoot down to the ground, the rearfoot must pronate. Physiologic tibia varum persists until 2 years of age, at which time it slowly changes to become genu valgum. This condition, too, encourages pronation. The proposed mechanism is movement of the center of gravity to the medial side of the weight-bearing foot, but there may be other explanations for it.

Primary ankle valgus is frequently overlooked in the workup of flatfoot. The exact incidence is unknown but, if overlooked, will result in error in control of the rearfoot because the pathology is proximal to the talocalcaneonavicular joint. In addition, orthoses cannot change this rigid and fixed eversion of the entire foot and ankle.

Talipes Calcaneovalgus

The position of talipes calcaneovalgus in the flatfoot spectrum has been largely ignored. The American College of Foot and Ankle Surgeons study failed to mention it.[36] Because of the use of the word talipes, it is grouped with the congenital foot and ankle deformities. It is included in several articles on congenital lower extremity deformities in infancy.[83–89] Some investigators believe that it spontaneously corrects.[46,72,90–92] Several investigators have studied its incidence in the population.[46,93] Nunes and Dutra[94] estimated the incidence at 4.2 per 10,000 live births.

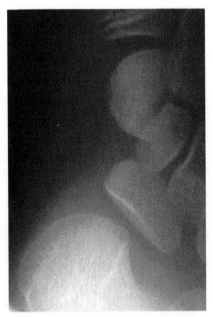

Fig. 7. As a consequence of attempting to compensate for severe ankle equinus, the talonavicular joint has transversely subluxed.

Its clinical appearance is distinctive. The foot is maximally dorsiflexed at the ankle so that the dorsum of the foot may make contact with the anterior tibia. The talocalcaneonavicular joint complex is maximally pronated. The forefoot is abducted. The anterior compartment muscles may be contracted. Although it is semiflexible, there is some resistance to full passive supination on manipulation. It is often associated with breech deliveries. Developmental hip dislocation and knee extension deformities are common.[95]

The differential diagnosis includes posteromedial bow deformity[96,97] and congenital convex pes valgus.[98] If there is a pure calcaneus deformity, it is necessary to verify that there is S1 function to exclude a paralytic deformity caused by myelomeningocele and other neurologic issues.[99] Examination of the contour of the tibia will help exclude posteromedial bow, but radiographs are often necessary (**Fig. 8**). Congenital convex pes valgus is similar to talipes calcaneovalgus. One key difference is the extreme rigidity in congenital convex pes valgus. The radiographic distinction is easily made. On lateral studies of calcaneovalgus deformity, the ankle is in a calcaneus position, whereas in congenital convex pes valgus the rearfoot is in equinus (**Fig. 9**).

The calcaneus ankle position spontaneously corrects or is treated by serial casting. The hyperpronation of the talocalcaneonavicular joint complex persists in untreated infants.

Oblique talus deformity was described by Kumar and colleagues.[37,38] Two types were described, depending on the position of the calcaneus. In 1 form, the calcaneal inclination angle is preserved and the talus is deviated significantly downward. In the second type, the talus is angled downward and the calcaneal inclination angle is reversed (**Fig. 10**). Oblique talus deformity may be persistence of the talocalcaneonavicular hyperpronation of talipes calcaneovalgus deformity.

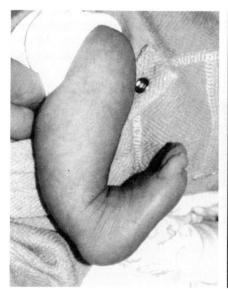
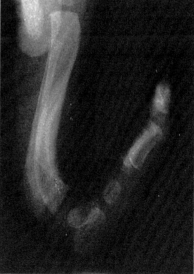

Fig. 8. An infant with posteromedial bow deformity could be mistaken for talipes calcaneovalgus or congenital convex pes valgus. The radiograph clearly demonstrates a posteromedial bow.

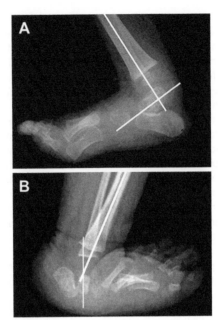

Fig. 9. Calcaneovalgus deformity is recognized radiographically on lateral view. (*A*) The ankle is in a calcaneus position with the talus dorsiflexed in the ankle mortise. (*B*) In congenital convex pes valgus, the talus is in a maximally plantarflexed position, and the ankle is in equinus.

DISCUSSION

Pediatric flatfoot is more than just a low arch. It is a complex condition of the rearfoot that may or may not be pathologic. Several subsets can be identified. Types such as congenital convex pes valgus (congenital vertical talus), flatfoot associated with tarsal coalitions, skewfoot deformity, flatfoot complicated by traumatic or iatrogenic

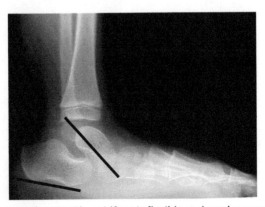

Fig. 10. Oblique talus deformity. The midfoot is flexible and can be manually reduced. The talus if plantarflexed at the talonavicular joint and the calcaneal inclination angle is reversed.

arthrosis, and flatfoot associated with systemic disease are clearly not physiologic. There is little argument that these will require some form of treatment. Their natural history tends more toward worsening, development of symptoms, and secondary joint changes over time. There are no data to suggest that they improve over time.

The issue of flexible flatfoot is another matter. There is little supportive evidence that it improves or worsens over time, therefore it is difficult to explain why there is so much polarization and contradiction when groups discuss biomechanical theory, what constitutes normal and abnormal, what is and is not deformity, and, especially, the pros and cons of treatment.[2,100–103]

As in the management of any other disease, treatment of flexible flatfoot should be goal-oriented. To be successful, there has to be a reasonable expectation that the goals can, and will, be met. Relief of clinical symptoms, positive modification of the natural history, and prevention of future complications are all laudable goals. However, their achievement remains scientifically unverifiable. There is room in evidence-based medicine to consider medicine-based evidence. Most people who attempt to manage flexible flatfoot in childhood will affirm that the clinical symptoms of plantar arch pain, leg fatigue, and even possibly the nocturnal pain syndrome respond to the use of orthotics. The real question is whether anything short of surgical reconstruction truly modifies the natural history. As an offshoot of that question, can extensive surgical intervention be justified for asymptomatic, or marginally symptomatic, flexible flatfoot?

Well-designed valid studies of the natural history of flexible flatfoot and the effects of modification of the natural history of flexible flatfoot are needed. There are some impediments to the design and execution of such studies. Assessment is made by clinical examination of ranges of motion, imaging, gait analysis, and subjective survey instruments. Interobserver and intraobserver reliability of clinical measurement of range of motion must be addressed. At present, imaging seems to be limited to the study of footprints and radiographic imaging. Formal gait-laboratory studies can be incorporated, but they are time consuming and expensive.

Radiographic imaging needs to be considered more carefully than it has been in the past. Several studies have used radiographic parameters for their conclusions on the diagnosis, natural history, and effects of treatment.[8,43,56,65,67–71] Measurements of the various angles assign a numerical value to the positional relationship of individual bones. For the skeletally mature person, this is straightforward. For the skeletally immature, these measurements assign a numerical value to the positional relationships of the ossific nuclei embedded in the cartilage anlagen. The ossification center for the talus begins in the neck, and the body ossifies last.[48,49,51] The ossification center for the calcaneus is eccentrically located and is along its inferior surface in the distal two-thirds of the developing bone.[49,51] It is also located lateral to the midline.[49] Consequently, many of the so-called changes in angular measurements with age that have been used to document a corrective natural history may merely represent the progression of normal ossification while the bony interrelationships remains the same. A photomicrograph of a fetal specimen shows the interrelationship of the developing bones appearing normal (**Fig. 11**). The perspective changes when the ossification centers are inserted are shown in **Fig. 12**.

It may be almost impossible to design and implement a study of the natural history of flexible flatfoot and the effects of treatment. It would require a prospective study of a large controlled patient population. There would have to be strict guidelines for enrollment in the study. The subjects would have to be studied for at least 10 to 15 years. The biggest drawback to the study would be repetitive x-ray exposure to the children for the sole purpose of gathering data. As an example, in the 1944 to 1945 Royal Canadian Army Medical Corps study, all 3619 subjects had radiographs. It is

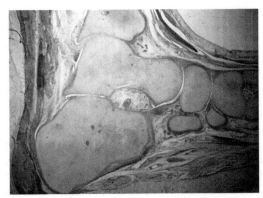

Fig. 11. Sagittal section of a fetal specimen (developmental age unknown) before the appearance of primary ossification centers. The overall alignment is anatomically correct.

unlikely that that could be done today. If treatment is included, there are only 2 possible hypotheses. The first is that treatment will not modify the natural history. Therefore, the study group will receive unnecessary treatment. The second is that treatment will modify the natural history, in which case the control group would not receive treatment that might prove beneficial. These issues raise serious moral and ethical concerns. It is unlikely that such a study would obtain Institutional Review Board approval.

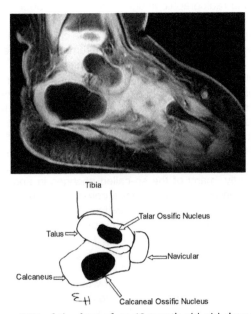

Fig. 12. Sagittal plane MRI of the foot of an 18-month-old girl shows the appearance of the primary ossification centers of the talus and the calcaneus as they relate to the cartilage anlagen. The ossification centers are drawn in relation to the primary cartilage anlagen.

SUMMARY

Those forms of flatfoot that are clearly pathologic are not controversial. The real issue is what to do with asymptomatic flexible flatfoot. It is hard to justify treating all forms of flexible flatfoot on the presumption that it will prevent pathologic conditions in adulthood, because there are no data to support that this actually happens. It is also hard to justify withholding treatment on the presumption that the condition will spontaneously correct, because the presence of flexible flatfoot in adolescence and adulthood proves that they do not all correct. Although not proven, one might be more confident in treating some of these conditions on the presumption that holding the foot in better alignment during rapid growth may prevent progression that may result from change in the developing bones secondary to remodeling during the endochondral ossification process. The same can be said for treating symptomatic flexible flatfoot, although the placebo effect of "doing something" remains unexplored.

Until supportive data are available, physicians must make judgments based on the situation at hand and their own personal experience. It would be wise to avoid the 2 extremes. The nihilistic approach of treating none of them is no better or worse than the approach that all flexible flatfoot is disease and needs forceful management. This statement is particularly true of aggressive surgical management involving ablation of motion segments. A course of action somewhere between the 2 extremes is more appropriate.

This overview of the history, causes, and pathophysiology of pediatric flatfoot can only be accomplished through literature search. A major drawback to this approach is the inability to guarantee recovery of all pertinent articles dealing with the topic. Such a search depends on identifying appropriate keywords. Therefore a possible limitation to this study is that certain important articles may have been omitted.

REFERENCES

1. Staheli LT. Evaluation of planovalgus foot deformities with special reference to the natural history. J Am Podiatr Med Assoc 1987;77(1):2–6.
2. Staheli LT. Planovalgus foot deformity. Current status. J Am Podiatr Med Assoc 1999;89(2):94–9.
3. Burns J, Keenan AM, Redmond A. Foot type and overuse injury in triathletes. J Am Podiatr Med Assoc 2005;95(3):235–41.
4. Manoli A 2nd, Graham B. The subtle cavus foot, "the underpronator". Foot Ankle Int 2005;26(3):256–63.
5. McCarthy DJ. The developmental anatomy of pes valgo planus. Clin Podiatr Med Surg 1989;6(3):491–509.
6. Greiner TM. The jargon of pedal movements. Foot Ankle Int 2007;28(1):109–25.
7. Huson A. Joints and movements of the foot: terminology and concepts. Acta Morphol Neerl Scand 1987;25(3):117–30.
8. Akcali O, Tiner M, Ozaksoy D. Effects of lower extremity rotation on prognosis of flexible flatfoot in children. Foot Ankle Int 2000;21(9):772–4.
9. Allen MK, Glasoe WM. Metrecom measurements of navicular drop in subjects with the anterior cruciate ligament injury. J Athl Train 2000;35(4):403–6.
10. Buchanan KR, Davis I. The relationship between forefoot, midfoot, and rearfoot static alignment in pain-free individuals. J Orthop Sports Phys Ther 2005;35(9):559–66.
11. Hargrave MD, Carcia CR, Gansneder BM, et al. Subtalar pronation does not influence impact forces or rate of loading during a single-leg landing. J Athl Train 2003;38(1):18–23.

12. Headlee DL, Leonard JL, Hart JM, et al. Fatigue of the plantar intrinsic foot muscles increases navicular drop. J Electromyogr Kinesiol 2008;18(3):420–5.

13. Hogan MT, Staheli LT. Arch height and lower limb pain: an adult civilian study. Foot Ankle Int 2002;23(1):43–7.

14. Holmes CF, Wilcox D, Fletcher JP. Effect of a modified, low-dye medial longitudinal arch taping procedure on the subtalar joint neutral position before and after light exercise. J Orthop Sports Phys Ther 2002;32(5):194–201.

15. Lange B, Chipchase L, Evans A. The effect of low-Dye taping on plantar pressures, during gait, in subjects with navicular drop exceeding 10 mm. J Orthop Sports Phys Ther 2004;34(4):201–9.

16. Leung AK, Cheng JC, Mak AF. Orthotic design and foot impression procedures to control foot alignment. Prosthet Orthot Int 2004;28(3):254–62.

17. Menz HB. Alternative techniques for the clinical assessment of foot pronation. J Am Podiatr Med Assoc 1998;88(5):253–5.

18. Mueller MJ, Host JV, Norton BJ. Navicular drop is a composite measure of excessive pronation. J Am Podiatr Med Assoc 1993;83(4):198–202.

19. Paton JS. The relationship between navicular drop and first metatarsophalangeal joint motion. J Am Podiatr Med Assoc 2006;96(4):313–7.

20. Radford JA, Burns J, Buchbinder R, et al. The effect of low-Dye taping on kinematic, kinetic and electromyographic variables: a systematic review. J Orthop Sports Phys Ther 2006;36(4):232–41.

21. Reinking MF. Exercise-related leg pain in female collegiate athletes: the influence of intrinsic and extrinsic factors. Am J Sports Med 2006;34(9):1500–7.

22. Reinking MF, Hayes AM. Intrinsic factors associated with exercise-related leg pain in collegiate cross-country runners. Clin J Sport Med 2006;16(1):10–4.

23. Schuh A, Honle W. [Pathogenesis of hallux valgus]. MMW Fortschr Med 2006;148(48):31–2 [in German].

24. Snook AG. The relationship between excessive pronation as measured by navicular drop and isokinetic strength of the anterior musculature. Foot Ankle Int 2001;22(3):234–40.

25. Trimble MH, Bishop MD, Buckley BD, et al. The relationship between clinical measurements of lower extremity posture and tibial translation. Clin Biomech (Bristol, Avon) 2002;17(4):286–90.

26. Vicenzino B, Griffiths SR, Griffiths LA, et al. Effects of anti-pronation tape and temporary orthotic on vertical navicular height before and after exercise. J Orthop Sports Phys Ther 2000;30(6):333–9.

27. Vicenzino B, Franettovich M, McPoil T, et al. Initial effects of the anti-pronation tape on the medial longitudinal arch during walking and running. Br J Sports Med 2005;39(12):939–43.

28. Vinicombe A, Raspovic A, Menz HB. Reliability of navicular displacement measurement as a clinical indicator of foot posture. J Am Podiatr Med Assoc 2001;91(5):262–8.

29. Whitford D, Esterman A. A randomized controlled trial of two types of in-shoe orthoses in children with flexible excess pronation of the feet. Foot Ankle Int 2007;28(6):715–23.

30. Green DR, Carol A. Planal dominance. J Am Podiatry Assoc 1984;74(2):98–103.

31. Labovitz JM. The algorithmic approach to pediatric flexible pes planovalgus. Clin Podiatr Med Surg 2006;23(1):57–76, viii.

32. Serrafian SK. Biomechanics of the subtalar joint complex. Clin Orthop Relat Res 1993;290:17–26.

33. Epeldegui T, Delgado E. Acetabulum pedis. Part I: talocalcaneonavicular joint socket in normal foot. J Pediatr Orthop B 1995;4(1):1–10.
34. Epeldegui T, Delgado E. Acetabulum pedis. Part II: talocalcaneonavicular joint socket in clubfoot. J Pediatr Orthop B 1995;4(1):11–6.
35. Golano P, Farinas O, Saenz I. The anatomy of the navicular and periarticular structures. Foot Ankle Clin 2004;9(1):1–23.
36. Harris EJ, Vanore JV, Thomas JL, et al. Diagnosis and treatment of pediatric flatfoot. J Foot Ankle Surg 2004;43(6):341–73.
37. Jayakumar S, Ramsey P. Vertical in the oblique talus: a diagnostic dilemma. Orthop Trans 1977;1:108.
38. Kumar SJ, Cowell HR, Ramsey PL. Vertical and oblique talus. Instr Course Lect 1982;31:235–51.
39. Harris EJ. The oblique talus deformity. What is it, and what is its clinical significance in the scheme of pronatory deformities? Clin Podiatr Med Surg 2000;17(3):419–42.
40. Jani L. [Pediatric flatfoot]. Orthopade 1986;15(3):199–204 [in German].
41. Zollinger H, Fellmann J. [Natural course of juvenile foot deformities]. Orthopade 1994;23(3):206–10 [in German].
42. Zollinger H, Exner GU. [The lax juvenile flexible flatfoot–disease or normal variant?] Ther Umsch 1995;52(7):449–53 [in German].
43. Harris RI, Beath T. Hypermobile flatfoot with short tendo Achilles. J Bone Joint Surg Am 1948;30:116–40.
44. Bahler A. [Insole management of pediatric flatfoot]. Orthopade 1986;15(3): 205–11 [in German].
45. Cappello T, Song KM. Determining treatment of flatfeet in children. Curr Opin Pediatr 1998;10(1):77–81.
46. Sullivan JA. Pediatric flatfoot: evaluation and management. J Am Acad Orthop Surg 1999;7(1):44–53.
47. Tax H. Conservative treatment of flatfoot in the newborn. Clin Podiatr Med Surg 1989;6(3):521–36.
48. Frisch H, Schmitt O, Eggers R. The ossification center of the talus. Ann Anat 1996;78(5):455–9.
49. Harris EJ. The relationship of the ossification centers of the talus and calcaneus to the developing bone. J Am Podiatry Assoc 1976;66(2):76–81.
50. Howard CB, Benson MK. The ossific nuclei and the cartilage anlage of the talus and calcaneum. J Bone Joint Surg Br 1992;74(4):620–3.
51. Hubbard AM, Meyer JS, Davidson RS, et al. Relationship between the ossification center and cartilaginous anlage in the normal hindfoot in children: study with MR imaging. AJR Am J Roentgenol 1993;161(4): 849–53.
52. Meyer DB, O'Rahilly R. The onset of ossification in the human calcaneus. Anat Embryol 1976;150(1):19–33.
53. Napolitano C, Walsh S, Mahoney L, et al. Risk factors that may adversely modify the natural history of the pediatric pronated foot. Clin Podiatr Med Surg 2000; 17(3):397–417.
54. Wenger DR, Mauldin D, Speck G, et al. Corrective shoes and inserts as treatment for flexible flatfoot in infants and children. J Bone Joint Surg Am 1989; 71(6):800–10.
55. Staheli L, Chew DE, Corbett M. The longitudinal arch. A survey of eight hundred and eighty-two feet in normal children and adults. J Bone Joint Surg Am 1987; 69(2):426–8.

56. Gould N, Moreland M, Alvarez R, et al. Development of the child's arch. Foot Ankle 1989;9(5):241–5.
57. Garcia-Rodriguez A, Martin-Jimenez F, Carnero-Varo M, et al. Flexible flat feet in children: a real problem? Pediatrics 1999;103(6):e84.
58. Lin CJ, Lai KA, Kuan TS, et al. Correlating factors and clinical significance of flexible flatfoot in preschool children. J Pediatr Orthop 2001;21(3):378–82.
59. El O, Akcali O, Kosay C, et al. Flexible flatfoot and related factors in primary school children: a report of a screening study. Rheumatol Int 2006;26(11):1050–3.
60. Pfeiffer M, Kotz R, Ledl T, et al. Prevalence of flat foot in preschool-aged children. Pediatrics 2006;118(2):634–9.
61. Forriol F, Pascual J. Footprint analysis between three and 17 years of age. Foot Ankle 1990;11(2):101–4.
62. Cowan DN, Jones BH, Robinson JR. Foot morphologic characteristics and risk of exercise-related injury. Arch Fam Med 1993;2(7):223–4.
63. Rudzki SJ. Injuries in Australian Army recruits. Part III: the accuracy of a pretraining orthopedics screen in predicting ultimate injury outcome. Mil Med 1997; 162(7):41–3.
64. Abdel-Fattah MM, Hassanin MM, Felembane FA, et al. Flat foot among Saudi Arabian army recruits: prevalence and risk factors. East Mediterr Health J 2006;12(1–2):211–7.
65. Kanatli U, Yetkin H, Cila E. Footprint and radiographic analysis of the feet. J Pediatr Orthop 2001;21(2):225–8.
66. Mickle KJ, Steele JR, Munro BJ. Is the foot structure of preschool children moderated by gender? J Pediatr Orthop 2008;28(5):593–6.
67. Harty MP. Imaging of pediatric foot disorders. Radiol Clin North Am 2001;39(4): 733–48.
68. Pehlivan O, Cilli F, Mahirogullari M, et al. Radiographic correlation of symptomatic and asymptomatic flexible flatfoot in young male adults. Int Orthop 2009; 33(2):447–50.
69. Kuhn DR, Shibley NJ, Austin WM, et al. Radiographic evaluation of weight-bearing orthotics and their effect on flexible pes planus. J Manipulative Physiol Ther 1999;22(4):221–6.
70. Vanderwilde R, Staheli LT, Chew DE, et al. Measurements on radiographs of the foot in normal infants and children. J Bone Joint Surg Am 1988;70(3):407–15.
71. Bleck EE, Berzins UJ. Conservative management of pes valgus with plantar flexed talus, flexible. Clin Orthop Relat Res 1977;Jan–Feb(122):85–94.
72. Wenger DR, Leach J. Foot deformities in infants and children. Pediatr Clin North Am 1986;33(6):1411–27.
73. Hefti F, Brunner R. [Flatfoot]. Orthopade 1999;28(2):159–72 [in German].
74. Li YH, Leong JC. Intoeing gait in children. Hong Kong Med J 1999;5(4):360–6.
75. Evans A. Relationship between "growing pains" and foot posture in children: single-case experimental designs in clinical practice. J Am Podiatr Med Assoc 2003;93(2):111–7.
76. Evans AM, Scutter SD. Are foot posture and functional health different in children with growing pains? Pediatr Int 2007;49(6):991–6.
77. Kirby KA. Subtalar joint axis location and rotational equilibrium theory of foot function. J Am Podiatr Med Assoc 2001;91(9):465–87.
78. McPoil T, Cornwall MW. Relationship between neutral subtalar joint position and pattern of rearfoot motion during walking. Foot Ankle Int 1994;15(3):141–5.
79. Ball KA, Afheldt MJ. Evolution of foot orthotics—part 2: research reshapes long-standing theory. J Manipulative Physiol Ther 2002;25(2):125–34.

80. Barroso JL, Barriga A, Barrecheguren EG, et al. [Congenital synostoses of the tarsus. Concept, classification, diagnosis and therapeutic approach]. Rev Med Univ Navarra 2001;45(1):43–52 [in Spanish].
81. Blakemore LC, Cooperman DR, Thompson GH. The rigid flatfoot. Tarsal coalitions. Clin Podiatr Med Surg 2000;17(3):531–55.
82. Lowy LJ. Pediatric peroneal spastic flatfoot in the absence of coalition. A suggested protocol. J Am Podiatr Med Assoc 1998;88(4):181–91.
83. Correll J, Berger N. [Diagnosis and treatment of disorders of the foot in children]. Orthopade 2005;34(10):1061–72 [quiz 1073–4] [in German].
84. Furdon SA, Donlon CR. Examination of the newborn foot: positional and structural abnormalities. Adv Neonatal Care 2002;2(5):248–58.
85. Gore AI, Spencer JP. The newborn foot. Am Fam Physician 2004;69(4):865–72.
86. Hart ES, Grottkau BE, Rebello GN, et al. The newborn foot: diagnosis and management of common conditions. Orthop Nurs 2005;24(5):313–21 [quiz 322–3].
87. Omololu B, Ogunlade SO, Alonge TO. Pattern of congenital orthopaedic malformations in an African teaching hospital. West Afr J Med 2005;24(2):92–5.
88. Sankar WN, Weiss J, Skaggs DL. Orthopaedic conditions in the newborn. J Am Acad Orthop Surg 2009;17(2):112–22.
89. Wynne-Davies R, Littlejohn A, Gormley J. Aetiology and interrelationship of some common skeletal deformities. (Talipes equinovarus and calcaneovalgus, metatarsus varus, congenital dislocation of the hip, and infantile idiopathic scoliosis). J Med Genet 1982;19(5):321–8.
90. Churgay CA. Diagnosis and treatment of pediatric foot deformities. Am Fam Physician 1993;47(4):883–9.
91. Hensinger RN. Rotational problems of the lower extremity. Postgrad Med 1976; 60(4):161–7.
92. Widhe T, Aaro S, Elmstedt E. Foot deformities in the newborn–incidence and prognosis. Acta Orthop Scand 1988;59(2):176–9.
93. Yu GV, Hladik J. Residual calcaneovalgus deformity: review of the literature and case study. J Foot Ankle Surg 1994;33(3):228–38.
94. Nunes D, Dutra MG. Epidemiological study of congenital talipes calcaneovalgus. Braz J Med Biol Res 1986;19(1):59–62.
95. Paton RW, Choudry Q. Neonatal foot deformities and their relationship to developmental dysplasia of the hip: an 11-year prospective longitudinal observational study. J Bone Joint Surg Br 2009;91(5):655–8.
96. Grimes JB, Blair VP 3rd, Gilula LA. Roentgen rounds #81. Posteromedial bowing of the tibia. Orthop Rev 1986;15(4):249–55.
97. Pappas AM. Congenital posteromedial bowing of the tibia and fibula. J Pediatr Orthop 1984;4(5):525–31.
98. Greenberg AJ. Congenital vertical talus and congenital calcaneovalgus deformity: a comparison. J Foot Surg 1981;20(4):189–93.
99. Rodrigues RC, Dias LS. Calcaneus deformity in spina bifida: results of anterolateral release. J Pediatr Orthop 1992;12(4):461–4.
100. Phillips RD. Planovalgus foot deformity revisited. J Am Podiatr Med Assoc 1999; 89(5):265–8 [author reply 269].
101. Root ML. Planovalgus foot deformity revisited. J Am Podiatr Med Assoc 1999; 89(5):268–9.
102. Evans AM. The flat-footed child—to treat or not to treat: what is the clinician to do? J Am Podiatr Med Assoc 2008;98(5):386–93.
103. Bresnahan P. Letter to the editor: the flat-footed child—to treat or not to treat. What is a clinician to do? J Am Podiatr Med Assoc 2009;99(2):178.

Equinus Deformity in the Pediatric Patient: Causes, Evaluation, and Management

Monique C. Gourdine-Shaw, DPM, LCDR, MSC, USN[a,b,c],
Bradley M. Lamm, DPM[c,*], John E. Herzenberg, MD, FRCSC[c],
Anil Bhave, PT[d,e]

KEYWORDS

- Equinus • Pediatric • External fixation
- Achilles tendon lengthening • Gastrocnemius recession
- Tendo-Achillis lengthening

Different body and limb segments grow at different rates, inducing varying muscle tensions during growth.[1] In addition, boys and girls grow at different rates.[1] The rate of growth for girls spikes at ages 5, 7, 10, and 13 years.[1] The estrogen-induced pubertal growth spurt in girls is one of the earliest manifestations of puberty. Growth of the legs and feet accelerates first, so that many girls have longer legs in proportion to their torso during the first year of puberty. The overall rate of growth tends to reach a peak velocity (as much as 7.5 to 10 cm) midway between thelarche and menarche and declines by the time menarche occurs.[1] In the 2 years after menarche, most girls grow approximately 5 cm before growth ceases at maximal adult height.[1] The rate of growth for boys spikes at ages 6, 11, and 14 years.[1] Compared with girls' early growth spurt, growth accelerates more slowly in boys and lasts longer, resulting in taller adult stature among men than women (on average, approximately 10 cm).[1] The difference is attributed to the much greater potency of estradiol compared with testosterone in

Two authors (BML and JEH) host an international teaching conference supported by Smith & Nephew.

[a] Medical Service Corps, United States Navy, United States Naval Academy, 250 Wood Road, Annapolis, MD 21402, USA

[b] Veterans Affairs Maryland Healthcare Systems, 10 North Greene Street, Baltimore, MD 21201, USA

[c] International Center for Limb Lengthening, Rubin Institute for Advanced Orthopedics, Sinai Hospital of Baltimore, 2401 West Belvedere Avenue, Baltimore, MD 21215, USA

[d] Rehabilitation, Rubin Institute for Advanced Orthopedics, Sinai Hospital of Baltimore, 2401 West Belvedere Avenue, Baltimore, MD 21215, USA

[e] Wasserman Gait Laboratory, Rubin Institute for Advanced Orthopedics, Sinai Hospital of Baltimore, 2401 West Belvedere Avenue, Baltimore, MD 21215, USA

* Corresponding author.

E-mail address: blamm@lifebridgehealth.org (B.M. Lamm).

Clin Podiatr Med Surg 27 (2010) 25–42

doi:10.1016/j.cpm.2009.10.003

0891-8422/09/$ – see front matter © 2010 Elsevier Inc. All rights reserved.

podiatric.theclinics.com

promoting bone growth, maturation, and epiphyseal closure. In boys, growth begins to accelerate approximately 9 months after the first signs of testicular enlargement.[1] The peak year of the growth spurt occurs approximately 2 years after the onset of puberty, reaching a peak velocity of approximately 8.5 to 12 cm of height per year.[1] The feet and hands experience the growth spurt first, followed by the limbs and then the trunk.[1] Epiphyseal closure in the upper and lower extremities occurs at approximately age 14 years for girls and 16 years for boys.[1] For 2 additional years, the remaining growth occurs in the axial skeleton (spine).[1]

During these periods of rapid growth, muscle contractures can occur, especially equinus deformity. Equinus is defined as the inability to dorsiflex the ankle enough to allow the heel to contact the supporting surface without some form of compensation in the mechanics of the lower limb and foot. During examination or assessment of children with equinus, it is important to understand the rates and intervals of rapid growth that may contribute to the equinus deformity.

The cause of pediatric ankle equinus may be primary or secondary. Primary equinus is caused by a pre-existing condition whereas secondary equinus develops from another cause. Equinus can be isolated, combined with other lower extremity deformities, or compensatory. In the pediatric population, congenital deformities, such as toe walking, Charcot-Marie-Tooth disease, cerebral palsy (CP), spina bifida, myelomeningocele, flatfoot, muscular dystrophy, arthrogryposis, fibular hemimelia, clubfoot, and limb length discrepancy, can produce equinus deformity. Acquired deformities from poliomyelitis, trauma, burns, and limb lengthening can also cause equinus. In adults, equinus can occur because of immobilization after trauma, lack of function of involved limb, or compensation for other conditions (**Box 1**).

It is important to distinguish between an equinus deformity and an equinus contracture. Equinus deformity is caused by an osseous condition that may or may not have soft tissue involvement whereas an equinus contracture is caused by only soft tissues (eg, tendons, ligaments, capsule, muscle, or fascia). Multiple factors may contribute to ankle equinus, including soft tissue (eg, posterior muscle group, ankle capsule, and subtalar joint) or bony deformities (eg, procurvatum and ankle osteophytes). Many types of equinus have been described in the literature, including osseous equinus, pseudoequinus (plantarflexed forefoot without ankle equinus), gastrocnemius equinus, gastrocnemius-soleus equinus, and a combination of types.[2]

PHYSICAL EXAMINATION AND RADIOGRAPHIC EVALUATION

Thorough evaluation of the pediatric foot is an essential portion of the examination. The purpose of the examination is to localize symptoms, identify dynamic and static mechanical abnormalities, and detect underlying disease states. Evaluation of major motor milestones determines whether a nervous system insult has occurred.[3,4] During the stance phase of gait, the greatest degree of dorsiflexion required is just before heel lift when the knee is maximally extended and the ankle must dorsiflex past perpendicular for smooth ambulation.[3,4] There is controversy in the literature as to the amount of dorsiflexion truly necessary for this to occur. It is better, therefore, to consider a normative range of values necessary for normal gait rather than a definitive number. The accepted range of normal ankle joint dorsiflexion is 3° to 15° past perpendicular with the knee extended.[2–4] When evaluating the negative influence of equinus on the limb, the method of compensation that a patient may exhibit is as important as the measurements of equinus and ankle joint dorsiflexion that are obtained during physical examination.

Patients may compensate for equinus deformity in many different ways and to varying degrees. The methods that patients use to compensate often determine which

Box 1
Examples of acquired and congenital equinus deformity
Acquired equinus
Poliomyelitis
Trauma
Burns
Limb lengthening
Lack of function of the involved limb
Compensation for other conditions
Congenital equinus
Cerebral Palsy
Charcot-Marie-Tooth disease
Spina bifida
Myelomeningocele
Flatfoot
Arthrogryposis
Clubfoot
Fibular hemimelia
Idiopathic toe walker
Muscular dystrophy

symptoms and pathologic conditions may coexist. Pronation of the subtalar joint with consequent unlocking of the oblique midtarsal joint axis, allowing for dorsiflexion and abduction to occur at the midfoot, constitutes fully compensated equinus. Common methods of compensation for equinus include forward torso lean, pelvic rotation, hip flexion, knee hyperextension, and external rotation of the leg. Therefore, patients can present with a variety of conditions, such as lower back pain, chondromalacia of the knee, Achilles tendinopathy, posterior tibial tendinopathy, painful flatfoot, plantar fasciitis, calcaneal apophysitis, Lisfranc's joint arthrosis, juvenile Charcot arthropathy, hallux valgus or rigidus, plantar ulceration, forefoot calluses, metatarsalgia, and hammertoe contractures.

The foot of an infant is malleable, which makes it difficult to distinguish between a temporary positional deformity and true structural deformity. Diagnosing equinus in this population requires knowledge of anatomy. Measuring a young child's ankle dorsiflexion, however, can help a physician diagnose primary equinus as the cause of flexible flatfoot, correction of which is essential for normal foot function.[1] Normal range of ankle dorsiflexion at age 3 years is 20° to 25°, diminishing to 10° by age 15.[2,3] The Silfverskiöld test helps a physician differentiate among gastrocnemius-soleus equinus, osseous equinus, soft tissue contracture, and soft tissue or osseous deformity (**Fig. 1**). Decreased ankle dorsiflexion during knee extension and flexion indicates gastrocnemius-soleus equinus whereas limited dorsiflexion with knee extended indicates only gastrocnemius equinus.[2,3] After the pathology of the equinus is determined and primary or secondary equinus is ruled out, treatment options may be determined.

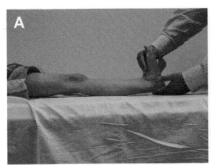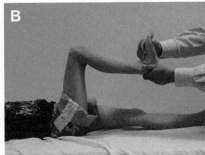

Fig. 1. (A) Clinical photograph of ankle dorsiflexion with knee extended (ie, part of the Silfverskiöld test). (B) Clinical photograph of ankle dorsiflexion with knee flexed (ie, part of the Silfverskiöld test). (Copyright 2009, Rubin Institute for Advanced Orthopedics, Sinai Hospital of Baltimore, Baltimore, MD.)

Radiography can be a critical tool in evaluation of pediatric foot abnormalities. The calcaneus usually starts to ossify by week 23 of gestation; the talus typically starts to ossify at approximately week 28.[5] At birth, only rounded ossific nuclei of some bones of the foot are visible radiographically.[5] Substantial portions of the calcaneus and talus usually are ossified by the first month of infancy.[5] The cuboid ossifies by 6 to 7 months of age, whereas the navicular ossifies between 9 months and 5 years of age.[5] The cuneiforms begin ossification between 3 months and 2.5 years of age, with the lateral cuneiform ossifying first. The metatarsals and phalanges are usually ossified at birth.[5] On average, many of the ossification centers appear on radiographs earlier in girls than in boys.[5]

Radiographic evaluation of the pediatric foot differs from radiographic assessment of the adult foot because radiographs of pediatric patients can contain less radiographic information secondary to variation in ossification. In addition, normative radiographic values for adults cannot necessarily be applied to the pediatric population because values tend to change with age.[6] Ultimately, radiographic studies can be used as an adjunct to clinical diagnosis of equinus and can be used to exclude other deformities.

Accurate diagnosis and assessment of equinus pose a challenge. Radiographs, with proper positioning and focus of the radiographic beam on the appropriate area of interest, are a valuable adjunct for accurate diagnosis of equinus deformities. Normal ranges and mean values of radiographic measurements of the pediatric foot change with age.[6] Inadequate dorsiflexion of the foot or significant equinus creates a falsely decreased talocalcaneal angle on the radiograph and should be clinically correlated when attempting to visualize the tibial and fibular shafts on the anteroposterior view. Lack of ankle dorsiflexion on lateral view radiographs may be secondary to improper positioning or an equinus deformity and also creates a falsely decreased talocalcaneal angle. During normal dorsiflexion, the range of the lateral talocalcaneal angle declines with age and is decreased with equinus or varus.[6] In maximum dorsiflexion, however, increases in the talocalcaneal and tibiocalcaneal angles occur with equinus or varus deformities. A radiograph showing maximum dorsiflexion also evaluates for anterior ankle bony block, which may produce equinus.

EQUINUS: ASSOCIATED CONDITIONS
Idiopathic Toe Walking

Toe walking is also known as habitual toe walking or congenital short Achilles tendon. The diagnosis is made by excluding all neuromuscular pathologies, especially when toddlers begin to walk. Toe walking may be considered normal when children begin to walk (until age 18 months). Normally, by 5 years of age, children have developed a stable heel-and-toe gait pattern, and by age 7 years, they usually have an adult gait pattern.[1,6] When children who are capable of heel-and-toe gait prefer to walk on their toes, it is considered habitual. Children with autism and attention-deficit hyperactivity spectrum disorders may have toe walking tendencies.[4,7] If untreated, idiopathic toe walking may lead to fixed contracture of the Achilles tendon and to valgus deformity of the hindfoot.[4,7]

Unilateral toe walking can be caused by limb length discrepancy, spastic equinus from stroke or hemiplegia, or Achilles tendon contracture. Common causes of bilateral toe walking include idiopathic toe walking and spastic diplegia. Bilateral toe walking is also associated with psychologic problems, such as autism and learning disorders. Late-onset bilateral toe walking can be attributed to multiple sclerosis, Charcot-Marie-Tooth disease, Duchenne's dystrophy, and spinal cord anomalies.

Muscular Dystrophy

Duchenne's dystrophy is a hereditary disease occurring only in boys and character-ized by progressive skeletal muscle weakness. Children with Duchenne's dystrophy seem normal at birth and have normal developmental milestones.[1] At approximately 3 years of age, they develop a tendency to fall.[1] Toe walking is compensatory early on and is necessary to maintain an upright posture. Usually, by age 5, the parents bring a child in for examination and there is a finding of pseudohypertrophy of the calf muscles, a positive Gowers sign, and toe walking because of an equinus contrac-ture of the calf muscles.[1]

Charcot-Marie-Tooth Disease

Charcot-Marie-Tooth disease is inherited as an autosomal recessive trait and is a common peripheral neuropathy involving the peroneal nerve in the lower extremity and the ulnar nerve in the upper extremity. The involvement is bilateral with one extremity affected more than the other; both extremities become progressively worse as a child grows. Weakness of the peroneal muscles with diminished deep tendon reflexes is noted.[1] The weak dorsiflexors force the recruitment of the long extensors to dorsiflex the foot during the swing phase.[1] Asymmetric muscle weakness leads to a cavus foot type with clawing of the toes that causes painful metatarsal heads and callus.[1] Shoe modification may benefit those with a mild deformity. Surgical correction of the cavus and claw toe deformities preserves function. The equinus in Charcot-Marie-Tooth disease is primarily forefoot rather than hindfoot equinus.[1]

Cerebral Palsy (Spastic Equinus)

CP is a result of a brain lesion (nonprogressive) with subsequent motor impairment. The four major classifications of CP describe different impaired movements: spastic, ataxic, flaccid, and athetoid. Spastic CP can be divided into three types. Children with hemiplegic spastic CP have dynamic equinus on the affected side and can be prescribed ankle-foot orthoses (AFOs) for prevention of equinus. Diplegic spastic CP is the most common type. These children are ambulatory with a scissor gait and flexed knees and hips of varying degrees (**Fig. 2**). Children with quadriplegic spastic CP usually do not walk because of the profound effects on all four limbs.

Children with CP walk at a later age than normal and do not adequately extend the knee during the swing phase of gait.[8,9] The deep tendon reflexes are hyperactive. Muscle contractures can worsen with time even though the underlying neurologic lesion is static and nonprogressive.[8,9] In children of preschool age, hemiplegic CP is

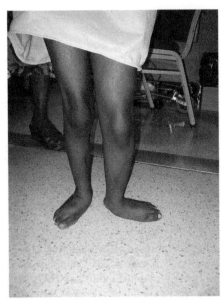

Fig. 2. Child with CP who has flatfoot, secondary to equinus, and midfoot break. (Copyright 2009, Rubin Institute for Advanced Orthopedics, Sinai Hospital of Baltimore, Baltimore, MD.)

suspected for asymmetric equinus, upper motor neuron syndrome, or sensory integration dysfunction for symmetric equinus.[8,9] The examination of equinus in athetoid CP is challenging, as it changes from moment to moment.

Spina Bifida (Spastic Equinus)

Spina bifida is the most common neural birth defect in the United States.[1] There are four types: occulta, closed neural tube defects, meningocele, and myelomeningocele. Occulta and closed neural tube defects rarely cause symptoms. Myelomeningocele can result in severe paralysis that prevents a child from walking. Multiple foot deformities occur including equinus, equinovarus, calcaneovalgus, cavovarus, varus, and calcaneus. Conservative measures, such as serial casting, often fail.[2,3] Soft tissue correction, including tendon releases or radical posteromedial release with Achilles tenotomy and plaster casting, is typically required.[2,3]

Equinus in Flatfoot

The phasic activity and function of the gastrocnemius muscle reach their peak at 50% to 60% of midstance of gait when the gastrocnemius muscle simultaneously flexes the knee and plantarflexes the ankle.[4,10] This is the moment when the maximum effect of an equinus deformity is noted. When a tight posterior muscle group is present, however, the foot or leg must compensate to maintain the foot securely on the ground. If a foot is able to compensate, the hindfoot severely pronates through the subtalar joint, allowing the midtarsal joint to unlock and dorsiflexion to increase through the oblique axis of the midtarsal joint. The degree of deformity depends on the foot type; some foot types are stable when affected by equinus whereas others are highly unstable (see **Fig. 2**). The lower limb compensates with hip flexion, lumbar lordosis, genu recurvatum, or persistent knee flexion to maintain the foot on the ground or to lift the heel off the ground early in the gait cycle. Function of the foot is compromised, and patients develop symptoms depending on their own method of compensation.[4]

Flexible flatfoot is the result of an equinus contracture whereas rigid flatfoot has a secondary equinus contracture because of the fixed foot position. At younger ages, the foot is more flexible and children weigh less, allowing the foot to withstand abnormal forces. As children age, however, their weight increases and the foot becomes less flexible. This causes compensation to be less tolerated and pain to ensue.

Osseous Equinus

Many types of osseous equinus exist and have contributing factors, including recurvatum of the tibia, forefoot equinus, flattop talus, anterior ankle osteophytes, forefoot cavus, trauma, and other congenital deformities. Radiographs should be used to evaluate the anterior and posterior ankle joint, the ankle joint morphology, the juxta-articular angles, and the overall foot and limb deformities to determine osseous involvement. Bony blocks from previous surgery or trauma of the anterior or posterior ankle can result in osseous equinus and painful impingement. When joint morphology is altered, as in a flattop talus, normal range of motion is not possible and equinus results. Pseudoequinus of forefoot cavus is an osseous foot deformity that results in a subsequent osseous equinus. Procurvatum deformity of the distal tibia may follow a partial growth arrest after trauma.

Clubfoot

In the United States, clubfoot occurs in 1 of 500 births. Idiopathic clubfoot is characterized by equinocavovarus and is the most common congenital deformity of the foot. During the initial examination, the idiopathic clubfoot has nonreducible equinus of the ankle, which is the characteristic presentation (**Fig. 3**). The initial treatment of clubfoot is the Ponseti method of serial casting.[11] The Ponseti method has proved successful in the correction of idiopathic clubfoot.[12–15] The equinus component is the last component of this deformity to be corrected and typically requires an Achilles tenotomy in 90% of cases.[12–15] When recurrence of clubfoot occurs, the first treatment is repeat casting using the Ponseti method. On occasion, a repeat tenotomy is required for recurrence in younger infants. For older infants or children, an open tendo-Achilles lengthening (TAL) with or without a posterior muscle group recession and or ankle/subtalar joint capsule release is required to correct recurrent equinus (**Fig. 4**).[12–15]

Arthrogryposis

Arthrogryposis is a syndrome that is characterized by contractures at birth. It can involve all four extremities and is often isolated to the distal extremities (ie, hands and feet). In the lower extremity, it is not uncommon for the hips to be flexed, abducted, and externally rotated with unilateral or bilateral hip dislocation.[16] The knees are in extension although flexion is possible. Children with arthrogryposis have a characteristic clubfoot deformity that rarely responds to serial casting or physical therapy.[16] Clubfoot associated with arthrogryposis is resistant to manipulation and casting and usually requires surgical correction. In this patient population, the Ponseti method of clubfoot casting[11] may provide initial correction of the deformity. Many cases relapse, however, and require open (eg, intra-articular and/or extra-articular release) or closed (eg, gradual correction with external fixation) surgical intervention.[16]

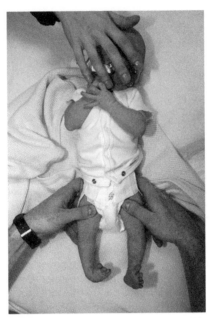

Fig. 3. Idiopathic right clubfoot with equinus, varus, forefoot cavus, and adduction. (Copyright 2009, Rubin Institute for Advanced Orthopedics, Sinai Hospital of Baltimore, Baltimore, MD.)

Fibular Hemimelia

Fibular hemimelia is the most common congenital limb deficiency in the lower extremity. It is characterized by a hypoplastic fibula, anterolateral bowing of the tibia, equinovalgus of the foot, tarsal coalition, short affected limb, absent tarsal bones or rays, ball-and-socket ankle, and syndactylization of digits (**Figs. 5–7**). Equinus is a powerful deforming force of the hypoplastic foot and ankle and thus causes severe foot and ankle deformities. Typically, fibular hemimelia is treated at multiple levels and

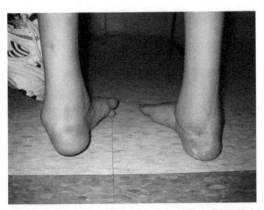

Fig. 4. Recurrent left clubfoot with cavoequinovarus. Note the incisions from previous surgical procedures. (Copyright 2009, Rubin Institute for Advanced Orthopedics, Sinai Hospital of Baltimore, Baltimore, MD.)

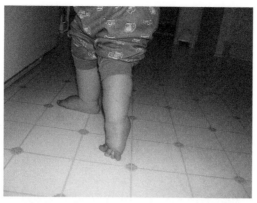

Fig. 5. Clinical photograph of a child with left fibular hemimelia. Note the short limb with equinus and the four toes. (Copyright 2009, Rubin Institute for Advanced Orthopedics, Sinai Hospital of Baltimore, Baltimore, MD.)

through various soft tissue procedures, including equinus correction and osseous procedures. Lengthening of the short bones exacerbates the tendency for equinus, necessitating concomitant releases.

CONSERVATIVE TREATMENT OF EQUINUS

Physical therapy, taping/strapping, orthoses, intramuscular injections, and serial casting are the conservative treatments that typically are used to combat equinus.

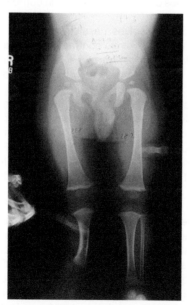

Fig. 6. Erect limb radiograph of an infant with right fibular hemimelia. Note the absent fibula, tibial bowing, and three metatarsals. (Copyright 2009, Rubin Institute for Advanced Orthopedics, Sinai Hospital of Baltimore, Baltimore, MD.)

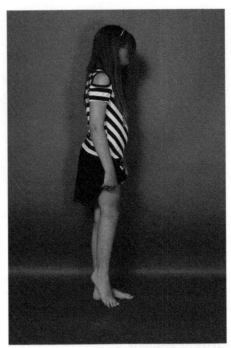

Fig. 7. Child with right fibular hemimelia and limb length discrepancy. Note the right equinus compensation for the limb length discrepancy. (Copyright 2009, Rubin Institute for Advanced Orthopedics, Sinai Hospital of Baltimore, Baltimore, MD.)

These conservative modalities can be used alone or in combination as the first stage of treatment.[10]

In general, physical therapy involves passive stretching exercises to prevent or delay hip flexion, hamstring, and equinus contractures because they can lead to the cessation of walking. Children can perform these exercises under the supervision of a therapist or parent. The goal is to enhance motor skills and maintain muscle length and flexibility.

Another option is kinesiotaping, which allows free joint movement without over-stretching adjacent muscles and is applied as a single layer of tape to improve circulation. The latex free elastic tape can be left in place for 3 to 5 days. The tape is applied along the length of the muscle as it is stretched. When applied at the insertion along the length of muscle to origin, the muscle relaxes or is inhibited. When applied at the origin along the length of muscle to insertion, the muscle is promoted to contract (**Fig. 8**).

Orthoses are beneficial to correct a flexible equinus deformity. An orthotic can be used for flexible flatfoot deformity to prevent excessive pronation caused by equinus. A contraindication for using an orthosis to control equinus is ankle range of motion that is restricted below neutral because a child is not able to achieve a plantigrade foot while wearing the orthosis. An isolated heel lift or an orthotic with a built-in heel lift can accommodate the equinus deformity, however. Skin ulceration and breakdown can occur when an orthosis is applied to a foot that excessively compensates for equinus. Skin ulceration or breakdown can also occur when a foot is insensate or patients are cognitively impaired and unable to report pain. Contractures must be reduced before fitting the AFO; any child who cannot achieve neutral ankle position cannot

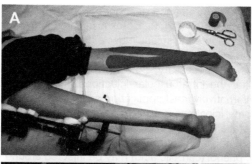

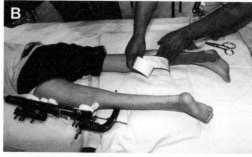

Fig. 8. Clinical photographs of kinesiotaping. (*A*) The latex free tape is applied in one layer, and the ends of the tape are rounded off before application. The tape is applied along the length of the muscle from insertion to origin as the muscle is stretched. When taping from insertion to origin, the muscle is encouraged to relax. Note that the tape may also be applied from the origin to the insertion, which will encourage the muscle to contract. (*B*) Leg is shown after kinesiotaping is applied. (Copyright 2009, Rubin Institute for Advanced Orthopedics, Sinai Hospital of Baltimore, Baltimore, MD.)

be braced.[4,10] An AFO can enclose the calf and should capture the leg just below the knee and include the foot to ensure control of the equinus deformity. Construction of the AFO may include restriction of ankle plantarflexion or ankle dorsiflexion assist. A prearticulated AFO can be made static and can be used by children until they have adequate tone reduction and can use the articulations. If children have severe hypertonia and no ankle range of motion, a solid AFO is prescribed. If there is no hypertonia and a physician suspects simple habitual toe walking, an articulated AFO can be used.

Botulinum toxin type A is a bacterial toxin produced by *Clostridium botulinum* that paralyzes the neuromuscular junction, which temporarily weakens the muscle. Botulinum toxin type A is the active ingredient in Botox (Allergan, Irvine, California). Although Botox is best known for its therapeutic use in CP, it can be used to treat equinus. Botox is best used to treat equinus deformities that result from dynamic contracture, a form of contracture that occurs when the muscle tension is so great that attempts at dorsiflexion fail.[17] Botox is injected into the overactive muscle rendering the muscle weaker for approximately 3 months; thus, injections may need to be repeated. High cost and the potential to develop antibodies against the toxin after repeat injections are disadvantages. Botox is reconstituted with 0.9% normal saline at a concentration of 100 U in 10 mL. Botox is administered to the gastrocnemius (medial and lateral heads) and soleus muscles at a dose of 10 U/kg of body weight.[17] The dosage should not exceed 12 U/kg (or 400 U) per visit or 50 U per injection site.[17]

Injection sites are identified using surface anatomy. General anesthesia or local anesthetic can be administered depending on the needs of the patient. Depending on the involvement of the soleus and gastrocnemius muscles, four sites on the calf muscle are injected with Botox (**Fig. 9**). Botox is injected into the superficial gastrocnemius muscle or deeper into the soleus muscle by pumping the syringe to distribute the medicine equally in different directions. Botox should not be injected into the vascular compartment. If necessary, Botox can be injected into the hip adductors and hamstrings. After the intramuscular injections, the leg is placed in a walking cast for 4 weeks. Alternatively, cast application can be delayed and the leg evaluated 1 to 2 weeks after the injections and, if necessary, the cast can be applied. If the contracture is myostatic in nature and causes the muscle to be permanently shortened, the only way to achieve joint motion is by lengthening the tendon.

As an alternative, phenol (carbolic acid) may be injected around the nerve carrying the exaggerated nerve signals to produce a similar kind of controlled time-bound muscle paralysis of a spastic muscle.[17] Only one or two injections can be administered for fear of scar formation on the nerve, whereas Botox may be used numerous times.

Equinus can be also be corrected by applying a series of casts that are changed weekly or biweekly. Placing a patient in a cast helps maintain improvement after manipulation. Application of casts should begin early in childhood to take advantage of the elasticity of contracted ligaments, joint capsules, and tendons. A long leg cast with the foot dorsiflexed to 90° and the knee extended provides the most stretch to the posterior muscle group. Short leg casts are not as effective in stretching the gastrocnemius muscle. Care should be taken not to cause cast sores or a rockerbottom foot deformity. At times, Botox is injected in combination with serial casting.

SURGICAL MANAGEMENT

Patients with isolated equinus or equinus as a component of a more complex deformity can undergo surgical treatment. Preoperative evaluation should include an assessment of whether multiple muscles in the lower extremities are involved.

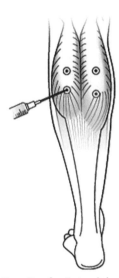

Fig. 9. Location of the four injection sites for Botox injection of the calf muscle. Botox can be injected superficially or deep into the gastrocnemius or soleus muscles as required based on the Silfverskiöld test. (Copyright 2009, Rubin Institute for Advanced Orthopedics, Sinai Hospital of Baltimore, Baltimore, MD.)

Evaluation of dorsiflexion with the knee straight and the knee flexed as described by the Silfverskiöld test is important to differentiate gastrocnemius equinus from gastrocnemius-soleus equinus. The Silfverskiöld test guides a surgeon's approach to correcting the equinus condition.

TAL, gastrocnemius recession, and gastrocnemius-soleus recession have been described to resolve equinus deformity. Each procedure has different advantages. As with any lengthening or tendon transfer, there is some residual deficit in the function of the muscle. Muscle recession has been shown to cause less muscle weakness than tendon lengthening.[2,3] The authors' have found, in their experience with children, less gastrocnemius-soleus weakness after gastrocnemius recession as compared with TAL.

Tendo-Achillis Lengthening

The most common operative procedure for the treatment of equinus is lengthening of the Achilles tendon. Multiple TAL procedures have been described for the correction of equinus deformity, including the Hoke, White, and Z lengthening procedures.[2,3] A percutaneous approach is used to reduce time in the operating room and the risk of delayed healing. Hoke[18] described a triple hemisection open TAL for triceps surae equinus. This procedure provides a reduced risk of rupture compared with the percutaneous approach but an increased risk of complication with delayed healing and hypertrophic scar formation. A surgeon usually performs the open TAL in the frontal plane, transecting the inferior fibers anteriorly and transecting the superior fibers posteriorly. Surgeons should be cautious not to overlengthen the tendon as this could result in profound weakness and dysfunction. Overlengthening is common when treating spastic equinus and, therefore, the authors prefer the Baumann (ie, gastrocnemius recession) procedure in which the soleus muscle is not as involved.

Gastrocnemius Recession

Many gastrocnemius recession procedures have been described in the literature, and each has its own risks and benefits. The Baumann procedure is performed proximally in the triceps surae muscle belly to treat equinus contracture (**Fig. 10**).[2,3] The incision is made two fingerbreadths from the medial border of the tibia. The crural fascia is then divided to expose the gastrocnemius muscle. Blunt dissection of the interval between the soleus muscle and gastrocnemius muscle is performed before dividing the plantaris tendon. The tendinous layer on the posterior surface of the gastrocnemius muscle is divided. It is important to identify the lateral-most edge of the gastrocnemius tendon. Next, tension is placed on the gastrocnemius muscle by dorsiflexing the ankle joint with the knee extended. A blade is used to make one transverse incision across the entire gastrocnemius muscle (gastrocnemius recession). The intermuscular septum between the medial and lateral heads of the gastrocnemius muscle also is carefully incised. After each recession, maximum ankle dorsiflexion is assessed clinically with the Silfverskiöld test. When two gastrocnemius recessions are indicated, the incisions are made 1 to 2 cm apart and are placed parallel to each other. Again, the ankle joint is manually dorsiflexed with the knee flexed and extended and, if desired, similar recessions can be made along the soleus muscle. The soleal cuts are placed distally to avoid overlapping the proximal gastrocnemius recession(s).[2]

One of the most common gastrocnemius recession techniques is the Baker[19] or reverse Baker,[4] in which the gastrocnemius tendon is lengthened in a tongue and groove fashion. Advantages of this technique include very controlled lengthening with sliding of the tendon to the appropriate length. The disadvantage, however, is that patients usually must be placed prone on the operating room table. This increases

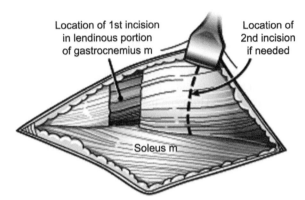

Location of 1st incision in lendinous portion of gastrocnemius m

Location of 2nd incision if needed

Soleus m

Fig. 10. Baumann procedure is performed through a mid-calf medial incision. Note the single incision across the gastrocnemius fascia (gastrocnemius recession). If increased dorsiflexion is needed, a second or third incision can be made with each incision placed 1 cm apart. m., muscle. (Copyright 2009, Rubin Institute for Advanced Orthopedics, Sinai Hospital of Baltimore, Baltimore, MD.)

surgical risk and necessitates turning patients to a supine position if a surgeon must perform other procedures. Another potential disadvantage is that surgeons usually perform this procedure slightly more inferior than the aponeurosis of the gastrocnemius muscle.

The Strayer procedure, described in 1950,[20] is a popular approach. The Strayer procedure involves lengthening of the gastrocnemius aponeurosis. The advantage of the Strayer procedure is that surgeons may perform it from a medial or posteromedial approach with patients in a supine position. This procedure isolates the gastrocnemius fibers with no soleal component. Since the procedure's rise in popularity, however, there has been an increase in the reported number of surgical or iatrogenic injuries to the sural nerve. The sural nerve pierces through the fascia in this area with some variability and is difficult to visualize on the lateral side of the gastrocnemius through the medial incision. The use of endoscopy for this procedure may aid in the visualization of the nerve, but the sural nerve remains at risk of injury with the Strayer or Baker technique.[21] The endoscopic gastrocnemius recession technique is limited in that the obturator and cannula instrumentation are straight whereas the structure that is to be lengthened (ie, the gastrocnemius) is round.

Gastrocnemius-Soleus Recession

The authors have found that the majority of children and adults present with combined gastrocnemius-soleus equinus. As an alternative to TAL, which weakens the entire triceps surae muscle, gastrocnemius-soleus recession is preferred. The authors do not perform gastrocnemius-soleus recession, to treat severe cases of contracture for which maximal lengthening is needed. Their technique is a modified form of the Vulpius technique[22] of gastrocnemius-soleus recession (**Fig. 11**). Under general anesthesia, patients are positioned supine with a thigh tourniquet. A 3-cm longitudinal midline incision is made at the most distal end of the soleus muscle. Careful dissection is then performed at that interval to identify the sural nerve and lesser saphenous vein. The tendon sheath is identified, and a longitudinal incision is made through it. The plantaris is identified and released. With the ankle dorsiflexed, the combined gastrocnemius and soleus tendons are cut transversely, stopping when the soleus muscle

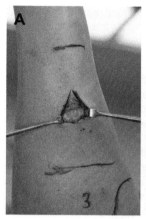
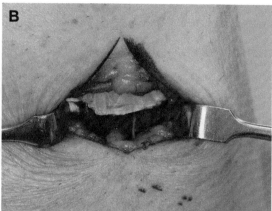

Fig. 11. Gastrocnemius-soleus recession. (*A*) A 3-cm longitudinal incision is made in the second anatomic level distal to the gastrocnemius aponeurosis. (*B*) A transverse incision is made through the combined gastrocnemius-soleus fascia stopping when the soleus muscle fibers are seen. The deep median raphe can be released if increased dorsiflexion is needed. (Copyright 2009, Rubin Institute for Advanced Orthopedics, Sinai Hospital of Baltimore, Baltimore, MD.)

fibers are seen. Then the ankle should be maximally dorsiflexed with the knee in full extension to separate the cut tendons (ie, recession). The Silfverskiöld test is again performed and if the equinus deformity is not completely corrected, the soleus tendon median raphe is identified and cut. The sheath covering the outer border of the tendon and skin is closed.

Other Procedures

Open ankle joint or subtalar joint releases may also be performed to release an equinus contracture. Early range of motion is critical otherwise stiffness may ensue. The authors prefer to avoid intra-articular releases if possible, holding true to the philosophy of Ponseti.[11]

Rehabilitation

Rehabilitation typically is dependent on which concomitant procedures were performed. In general, after undergoing a recession or TAL the leg is protected by placing it in a weight-bearing short leg cast or boot for 4 weeks. For 4 weeks at night, patients maintain the maximum stretch on the gastrocnemius muscle by using a knee immobilizer or keeping the foot on a pillow to extend the knee. Physical therapy is started 4 weeks after surgery.

Complications

The most common complications are recurrence of equinus deformity or overlengthening. The functional limitation created by overlengthening of the Achilles tendon is crouch or calcaneal gait. This occurs because of the inability of the weakened triceps surae muscle to restrain the forward movement of the tibia when the center of gravity moves in front of the ankle center of rotation during gait.[2,3] Because patients lose the normal plantarflexion or knee extension, the weight-bearing line becomes anterior to the ankle and hip center of rotation and posterior to the knee joint, resulting in flexion at the knee and hip with dorsiflexion of the ankle.[2,3] This causes secondary hip and knee flexion contractures and severe patellofemoral pain, which may lead to the cessation of walking. Weakening of the soleus muscle could also create knee instability.

EXTERNAL FIXATION

Gradual correction of the equinus deformity is an alternative to open procedures and is well tolerated in pediatric patients.[23] When large or open surgery has failed, gradual correction of equinus with external fixation (constrained or unconstrained) is preferred (**Fig. 12**). External fixation allows patients to ambulate when treating a complex and sometimes multiplanar deformity. The risk of adversely affecting the Blix contractile force curve as in tendon lengthening is largely avoided with distraction. Ilizarov distraction is the preferred method to correct stiff ankles, as performing repeat open surgery through extensive scar tissue formation is an overwhelming task. By using external fixation, the authors avoid procedures, such as talectomy and triple arthrodesis, that are disabling. In such cases, the joints typically are normal and the equinus that developed compensates for other deformities.[23]

At the authors' institution, the Ilizarov method is often used to correct clubfoot, equinus, supinated foot, pronated foot, hemimelia, arthrogryposis, and myelodysplastic deformity. The constrained frame allows patients to perform physical therapy whereas the Taylor Spatial Frame (Smith & Nephew, Memphis, Tennessee) and unconstrained constructs do not. Children younger than 8 years can undergo soft tissue and joint distraction, whereas children 8 years and older typically undergo distraction osteogenesis. Younger children undergo soft tissue and joint distraction because they still possess some degree of biologic plasticity (ie, remodeling potential) of their bones and cartilage.[1,4,23] The Ilizarov method of joint and soft tissue distraction is analogous to treating infants with serial casting. With casting, pressure is applied to the skin and the joints primarily experience compressive forces. In distinction, the Ilizarov method applies distraction forces across the joints. The stiff soft tissues are stretched rather than surgically released, avoiding extensive pericapsular and intra-articular fibrosis scarring.

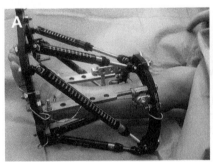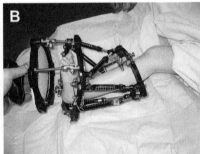

Fig. 12. (*A*) Clinical photograph obtained before correction. A 3-year-old girl with recurrent clubfoot had undergone prior open surgery. External fixation was applied for gradual soft tissue correction of the equinus and adductovarus. Note the talar neck wire is connected to the tibial ring for the adductovarus correction (first stage) about the subtalar joint. The ankle is in equinus. (*B*) Clinical photograph obtained after correction. Note the talar neck wire is connected to the foot ring for the equinus correction (second stage) about the ankle joint. The ankle is excessively dorsiflexed to allow for slight rebound of equinus. When full correction was obtained, the external fixator was maintained for 6 additional weeks. (Copyright 2009, Rubin Institute for Advanced Orthopedics, Sinai Hospital of Baltimore, Baltimore, MD.)

The foot should be overcorrected by 5° to 10° in the plane of correction because rebound of the soft tissues is predictable. The foot should be held in the overcorrected position for 4 to 6 weeks. Major corrections require control of the toes with slings, transverse wires, or longitudinal wires. After removal, a long leg cast is applied to maintain the overcorrected position. A custom molded AFO should be worn for the first 6 months. If dynamic recurrence is experienced, the appropriate tendon transfer should be considered. Rigid recurrences might require appropriate corrective osteotomies or arthrodesis.

The Ilizarov External Fixator (Smith & Nephew, Memphis, Tennessee) and Taylor Spatial Frame can also be used, in conjunction with the principles described by Ponseti,[11] for correction of equinovarus (ie, clubfoot) deformity (see **Fig. 12**). In the Ponseti sequence, the foot is first externally rotated through the subtalar joint. The initial correction with the Taylor Spatial Fame is programmed for external rotation, valgus correction, and minimal dorsiflexion. A lateral olive wire through the talar neck mimics the thumb that Ponseti uses for counterpressure. This wire is attached to the proximal tibial ring. Once the foot is externally rotated approximately 40°, the talus neck olive wire is connected to the foot ring to allow for dorsiflexion of the ankle. Next, an additional program is created to allow for ankle dorsiflexion and then the overcorrected position is maintained for 6 weeks. The combined correction of the subtalar and ankle joint (described previously) is called kinematic coupling.

SUMMARY

A thorough physical examination and radiographic analysis should be used to determine whether conservative or surgical treatment is the best option. The age of a patient, the cause of the deformity, and potential complications should also be considered. Typically, conservative treatment options are initially used to manage equinus. When conservative treatments are no longer effective, patients can undergo open or percutaneous surgical correction. For more complex deformities, gradual correction with external fixation may be the best option.

ACKNOWLEDGMENTS

The authors would like to thank Amanda Chase, MA, for her expeditious editing of this manuscript; Roland Starr, MS, for his assistance; Joy Marlowe, MA, for her illustrative expertise; and Joe Michalski, MA, for his expert photography.

REFERENCES

1. Tachdjian M.O. Atlas of pediatric orthopedic surgery, vol. 21. 1st edition. Philadelphia: W.B. Saunders Company; 1994.
2. Herzenberg JE, Lamm BM, Corwin C, et al. Isolated recession of the gastrocnemius muscle: the Baumann procedure. Foot Ankle Int 2007;28(11):1154–9.
3. Lamm BM, Paley D, Herzenberg JE. Gastrocnemius soleus recession: a simpler, more limited approach. J Am Podiatr Med Assoc 2005;95(1):18–25.
4. Banks AS, Downey MS, Martin DE, et-al. McGlamry's comprehensive textbook of foot and ankle surgery, vol. 1. 3rd edition. Philadelphia: Lippincott Williams & Wilkins; 2001.
5. Katz MA, Davidson RS, Chan PSH, et al. Plain radiographic evaluation of the pediatric foot and its deformities. University of Pennsylvania Orthopaedic Journal 1997;10:30–9.

6. Vanderwilde R, Staheli LT, Chew DE, et al. Measurements on radiographs of the foot in normal infants and children. J Bone Joint Surg Am 1988;70(3):407–15.
7. Stricker SJ. Evaluation and treatment of the child with tiptoe gait. International Pediatrics 2006;21(2):91–9.
8. Tachdjian MO. The child's foot. Philadelphia: W.B. Saunders Company; 1985.
9. Morrissy RT, Weinstein SL. Lovell and winter's pediatric orthopaedics, vol. 1. 4th edition. Philadelphia: Lippincott–Raven Publishers;1996.
10. Valmassay R. Biomechanical evaluation of the child. In: Valmassay R, editor. Clinical biomechanics of the lower extremity. St. Louis (MO): Mosby; 1996. p. 244–7.
11. Ponseti IV. Congenital clubfoot: fundamentals of treatment. New York: Oxford Univerisity Press Inc; 1996.
12. Lamm BM, Herzenberg JE. Ponseti method revolutionizes clubfoot treatment. BioMechanics 2005;12(10):47–58.
13. Ranade A, Lamm BM, Herzenberg JE. A review article: Ponseti method for the treatment of idiopathic clubfoot. J Foot and Ankle Surgery (India) 2006;21(1):1–8.
14. Herzenberg JE, Radler C, Bor N. Ponseti versus traditional methods of casting for idiopathic clubfoot. J Pediatr Orthop 2002;22(4):517–21.
15. Bor N, Herzenberg JE, Frick SL. Ponseti management of clubfoot in older infants. Clin Orthop 2006;444:224–8.
16. Tolo VT, Wood B. Pediatric orthopaedics in primary care. Baltimore (MD): Williams & Wilkins; 1993.
17. Graham HK, Aoki KR, Autti-Rämö I, et al. Recommendations for the use of botulinum toxin type A in the management of cerebral palsy. Gait Posture 2000;11(1):67–79.
18. Hoke M. An operation for the correction of extremely relaxed flat feet. J Bone Joint Surg Am 1931;13:773–83.
19. Baker LD. A rational approach to the surgical needs of the cerebral palsy patient. J Bone Joint Surg Am 1956;38:313–23.
20. Strayer LM Jr. Recession of the gastrocnemius: an opportunity to relieve spastic contracture of the calf muscles. J Bone Joint Surg Am 1950;32:671.
21. Saxena A, Gollwitzer H, Widtfeldt A, et al. [Endoscopic gastrocnemius recession as therapy for gastrocnemius equinus]. Z Orthop Unfall 2007;145(4):499–504 [in German].
22. Vulpius O, Stoffel A. Tenotomie der end schnen der mm. gastrocnemius el soleus mittels mittels rutschenlassens nach vulpius. In: Vulpius O, Stoffel A, editors. Orthopadische Operationslehre. Stuttgart (Germany): Verlag von Ferdinand Enke; 1913. p. 29–31.
23. Lamm BM, Standard SC, Galley IJ, et al. External fixation for the foot and ankle in children. Clin Podiatr Med Surg 2006;23(1):137–66, ix.

Clinical Diagnosis and Assessment of the Pediatric Pes Planovalgus Deformity

Nitza Rodriguez, DPM[a],*, Russell G. Volpe, DPM[b]

KEYWORDS

- flatfoot • Pediatric flatfoot • Pes planovalgus
- Coalition • Calcaneovalgus

Pediatric flatfoot is considered to be either congenital or acquired with flexible and rigid categories. Flexible flatfoot is characterized by the presence of a normal arch nonweight bearing and a lowered arch on weight bearing, and it may be present with or without symptoms. Rigid flatfoot has a markedly reduced range of motion non-weight bearing with a lowered arch in all positions; it is more frequently associated with underlying pathology that should be investigated thoroughly.[1]

Although it has been reported that most children will achieve partial spontaneous correction of their flatfoot, it also has been demonstrated through gait analysis that children with flatfeet walk slower and perform physical activities poorly compared with children without flatfeet.[2,3] Various studies have concluded that the prevalence of flatfoot is influenced by multiple factors: age, height, weight, gender, genu valgum, and joint laxity.[3–5] Pheffer and colleagues reported a decrease in prevalence with increasing age and a higher prevalence of flatfeet in boys (52%) than in girls (36%) when evaluating a group of 3- to 6-year-old children.[4] A study of foot anthropometry (arch index derived from plantar footprints and midfoot plantar fat pad thickness measured by ultrasound) found that preschool boys displayed significantly flatter feet than girls. They attributed the increased incidence of flat-footedness in boys to the thicker fat pad in the medial midfoot, however, and further suggested that the development of the medial longitudinal arch may be progressing at a slower rate in boys than in girls.[6]

[a] Northern California Foot and Ankle Center, 45 Castro Street Suite # 315, San Francisco, CA 94114, USA
[b] Department of Orthopedics and Pediatrics, New York College of Podiatric Medicine, Foot Clinics of New York, 53-55 East 124th Street, New York, NY 10035, USA
* Corresponding author.
E-mail address: nitzarodriguez@gmail.com (N. Rodriguez).

Clin Podiatr Med Surg 27 (2010) 43–58
doi:10.1016/j.cpm.2009.08.005
0891-8422/09/$ – see front matter © 2010 Elsevier Inc. All rights reserved.

podiatric.theclinics.com

THE HISTORY

The careful evaluation of the pediatric flatfoot begins with a detailed history. This should start with the age of onset, because many underlying conditions may be age-specific.[7] Presence or absence of symptoms, location of pain, and when pain occurs may contribute to the diagnosis. A painful flatfoot off weight bearing may be indicative of inflammatory arthritis, infection, or possibly a bone tumor.[7] Flatfeet that persist over time or show signs of clinical progression are generally of greater consequence. Symptoms may include pain in the foot, leg, and knee, or be related to posture. Children may not complain of pain, however, but report decreased endurance or voluntary withdrawal from physical activity and sports. Additional inquiries include family history, history of trauma, gestational history, developmental milestones, and associated medical conditions.[1,7-9] Other factors such as obesity, neuromuscular disorders and superstructural deformities above the ankle as comorbidities are important in determining the significance of an individual flatfoot.[1,3-5,7,10] This detailed medical history, along with a review of systems, may identify previously unsuspected medical conditions.

THE PHYSICAL EXAMINATION

An organized systematic physical examination including gait analysis and both weight bearing and off weight bearing lower extremity biomechanical examinations are key in diagnosis of a pediatric flatfoot. Gait analysis should be observed with both the child barefoot and wearing shoes. Abnormal pronation may be masked walking in supportive shoes, leading to a false negative.[11]

Gait assessment begins with the patient walking and a simple visual observation of whether the gait pattern is normal, antalgic, or indicative of neuromuscular disease.[1,7,12] Overall observational analysis should include basic components of head and shoulder position, arm position and swing, pelvic height in stance, symmetry, and length of step and the relationship of foot to the leg. In the swing phase of gait, one should note the quality and length of leg swing and the flexion/extension positions of the hip, knee, and ankle.[11] The angular deviation of the foot from the line of progression should be assessed. Care should be taken to observe foot contact position (heel first or midfoot or forefoot contact, medial or plantar prominence of the medial midfoot, and position of the calcaneus in the frontal plane at contact and after heel lift).[1,11]

The child also should be asked to walk up and down a hallway demonstrating both toe walking and heel walking. Subtle asymmetries in these gait patterns may unmask neurologic or musculoskeletal disorders. If the medial longitudinal arch is absent with the patient standing still, the examiner should focus on the reconstitution of the arch on toe rise.[7,11] Important characteristic findings that are observed in the pediatric pes valgus gait consist of a maximally pronated subtalar joint throughout midstance and propulsion, eversion of the subtalar joint after heel lift, abducted angle of gait, and shortened stride length with poor-quality propulsion.

A comprehensive biomechanical examination of the lower extremity should begin at the hip when assessing a pediatric patient with a flatfoot. Rotation of the child's hip in an extended and flexed position to evaluate transverse range of motion should be performed, evaluating for femoral anteversion or internal femoral position. Marking the patellar position to serve as a reference for rotation of the femoral head in the acetabulum is a useful method (**Fig. 1**). The "hands-on-a-clock" method is a helpful way to quantify the degree of rotation in each direction at the hip.

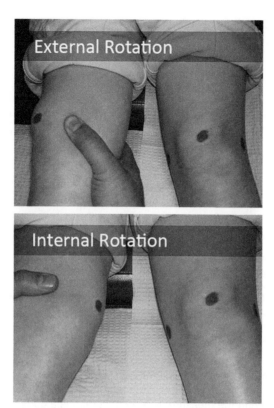

Fig. 1. Demonstrates external/internal rotation of the hip. Note the patellar marking to serve as a reference for rotation of the femoral head in the acetabulum. The hands-on-a-clock method is a helpful way to quantify the degree of rotation in each direction at the hip.

True femoral torsion, femoral antetorsion, the osseous twist of the long axis of the femur in the transverse plane, are evaluated best clinically using Ryder's test, which places the greater trochanter of the femur parallel to the frontal plane of the child while lying supine. (**Fig. 2**) With the proximal segment maintained in this position parallel to the frontal plane, the transcondylar axis of the femur is evaluated at the level of the knee joint. The normal newborn has approximately 30° of internal femoral torsion, which reduces with growth to an internal angle of about 10° by skeletal maturity.[13,14]

Transverse plane knee joint motion is assessed by stabilizing the femur and rotating the tibiofibular segment internally and externally. There is approximately 10° to 15° of motion at the knee joint in the normal newborn, which reduces to nearly zero by about 1 year of age. Internal tibial torsion is assessed clinically by placing the knee joint (femoral condyles) on the frontal plane and using the patella (marking the center of the patella is helpful) as a reference for the midpoint of the two condyles. Condylar placement on the frontal plane is accomplished by aligning the patella with the midpoint of the transverse plane, placing it so it is pointing upward. Once the condyles are placed and held in the frontal plane, the transmalleolar axis of the distal tibia and fibula is evaluated. Goniometers, tractographs, and other angular measuring devices are useful for quantifying this alignment. If the transmalleolar axis is parallel to the frontal plane, then a malleolar angle of 0° is assessed. If the lateral malleolus is posterior to the frontal plane (and to the medial malleolus), then an external malleolar angle

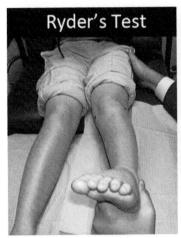
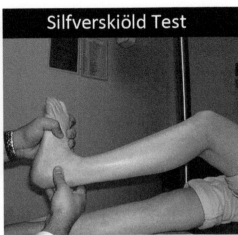

Fig. 2. Ryder's & Silfverskiöld test. Ryder's test assesses femoral antetorsion by placing the greater trochanter of the femur parallel to the frontal plane of the child while lying supine. With the proximal segment maintained in this position parallel to the frontal plane, the transcondylar axis of the femur is evaluated at the level of the knee joint. Note the examiner's right hand locating the greater trochanter. Silfverskiöld test assesses dorsiflexion of a neutral foot on the lower leg with the knee extended (testing gastrocnemius) and knee flexed (testing soleus or bony block).

is present, and the degree of external rotation is measured. Care must be taken to ensure that the femoral condyles remain in the frontal plane (as marked by a central patellar position) during the measurement procedure. It is a common error in clinical assessment to externally rotate the femur and thus the condyles, creating a falsely external malleolar angle, obscuring true internal tibial torsion when it is present. The normal malleolar angle in a newborn is approximately 0°, increasing to an external angle of 5° to 8° by age 1 year, 9° by 18 months, and increasing an additional 2° external per year after that until reaching a mature malleolar angle of 13° to 18° external by age 6 to 7 years.[15,16]

A thorough evaluation of the sagittal plane alignment of the child's lower extremity should be undertaken to identify any muscular restriction or bony limitation (equinus influences) that may lead to compensations in the midsagittal plane. Equinus influences in the superstructure may be found beginning proximally with tight hip flexor muscles identified with a Thomas test. In a supine examination, flexion of one hip to the torso should allow the contralateral hip to remain in a fully extended position. Rising of the contralateral leg after this flexion maneuver on the opposite limb is a clinical sign of hip flexor tightness. Next, the child should be checked for tightness of the hamstring muscles on straight-leg raise, popliteal angle, or toe-touching examination.

Equinus is identified at the ankle joint. The gastrocnemius and soleus muscles act on the ankle joint, and a minimum of 5° of ankle dorsiflexion is required for normal anterior movement of the tibia and fibula over the planted foot during midstance phase of gait. The appropriate clinical examination is the Silfverskiold test to assess dorsiflexion of a neutral foot on the lower leg with the knee extended (testing gastrocnemius) and knee flexed (testing soleus or bony block) **(Fig. 2)**.

The resting calcaneal stance position (RCSP) and the neutral calcaneal stance position (NCSP) should be measured for comparison. The RCSP is assessed while the patient is standing in his or her normal angle and base of gait. The patient's hindfoot position is assessed posteriorly with a line that bisects the calcaneus with reference to the midsagittal plane (**Fig.** 3A). The NCSP is assessed in a similar fashion but with the subtalar joint placed in neutral position. In RCSP, the child is asked to lift the lateral forefoot as much as possible without knee flexion, and if less than 2° of additional eversion are seen, then RCSP is considered maximally pronated. The child then is told to stand in angle and base of gait without any attempt to move or raise the arch. The examiner's fingers are placed plantar to the medial navicular to gauge resistance to subtalar joint (STJ) supination by digital force applied to the STJ axis.

Bisecting the calcaneus and maximally inverting and everting the subtalar joint relative to the distal one third of the leg assess the subtalar joint motion. The amount of subtalar joint range of motion is much greater in a child than an adolescent or adult; however the 2:1 ratio of inversion-to-eversion is maintained.[17]

Assessing the forefoot-to-rearfoot relationship is necessary to identify any frontal plane foot types with compensatory subtalar joint pronation. This is accomplished with the child in a prone position and the calcaneus properly bisected. Placing a dorsiflexory force on the plantar surface of the fifth metatarsal to resistance locks the midtarsal joint, and the subtalar joint should be maintained in neutral position (**Fig.** 3B). In a rectus foot type, the plane of the metatarsals should be perpendicular to the bisection of the rearfoot.[17]

It is also important to assess the hypermobility of the medial column by placing the subtalar joint in neutral and loading the lateral metatarsals with one hand while evaluating the first ray motion. Other diagnostic maneuvers should include the Hubscher maneuver or great toe test of Jack.

Characteristic physical findings in the pediatric flatfoot will vary with age and type of flatfoot. Some characteristic findings may include altered gait, equinus, calcaneal valgus, decreased medial longitudinal arch structure, medial talar head prominence, hypermobility, and the presence of calluses (**Fig.** 4).[1,7,18–20] Specifically, common clinical features of an acquired flexible flatfoot are:

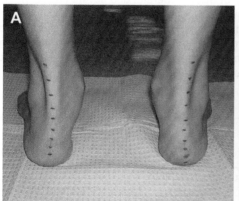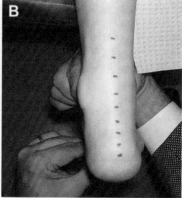

Fig. 23. (A) The resting calcaneal stance position is assessed while the patient is standing in normal angle and base of gait. (B) Frontal plane forefoot-to-rearfoot relationship with the child in a prone position and the calcaneus properly bisected. Placing a dorsiflexory force on the plantar surface of the fifth metatarsal to resistance locks the midtarsal joint with the subtalar joint maintained in neutral position.

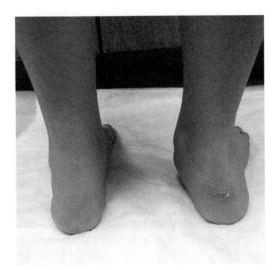

Fig. 4. Demonstrating characteristic findings in a pediatric pes planovalgus foot type. Note the significant calcaneal valgus with a decreased medial longitudinal arch structure and the medial talar head prominence.

Everted calcaneus
Medial talar head prominence
Transverse plane abduction of midfoot
Collapse of the medial longitudinal arch
Hypermobility
Pronated gait equinus

Other clinical findings are tenderness on palpation along the medial column, metatarsal heads, plantar fascia, sinus tarsi and ankle.[1]

In asymptomatic cases of pediatric pes planovalgus, some of the physical characteristics can be quantified in a system of mild, moderate, and severe (**Table 1**). The senior author's (RGV) approach is any child with two of the three clinical findings graded as moderate or severe should be treated with or without symptoms. Two of these three clinical criteria graded as moderate or higher indicate significant evidence of acquired pes planovalgus, and presence of these criteria may serve as a useful guide for when treatment should be recommended.

Table 1
Volpe's treatment classification system

	Mild	Moderate	Severe
Collapse of medial arch	Collapsed but arch is visible	Not visible	Not visible, convexity noted from talar head
RCSP (children >7 y)[a]	2°–5° valgus	6°–10° valgus	>10° valgus
Too many toes sign	Toes 4 & 5	Toes 3–5	Toes 2–5

Based on these quantifications, a system was devised for determining when to recommend treatment in a child with an asymptomatic acquired flexible pes valgus.
[a] For children younger than 7 years, use 8 – (age of child) = Maximum RCSP normal for age.[41]

DIAGNOSTIC STUDIES

Various imaging studies to help in diagnosis may include radiographs (weight-bearing), magnetic resonance imaging (MRI), computed tomography (CT), and bone scans.[1,7,18,19,21–23] **Table 2** provides common radiographic parameters used to evaluate pediatric pes planovalgus. Serologic studies may be useful in differentiating symptoms associated with inflammatory diseases and those originating from faulty biomechanics leading to overuse symptoms.[1,7] Footprint analysis may be used effectively as screening studies.[24]

DIAGNOSIS AND CATEGORIZATION OF FLATFOOT
Congenital Flexible Flatfoot

Calcaneovalgus
Congenital calcaneovalgus (CCV) is a flexible deformity that is usually present at birth (**Fig. 5**).[18] It is found more commonly in females and can be unilateral or bilateral (**Figs. 6** and **7**). When dealing with CCV, it is important to inquire about any associated abnormalities or neuromuscular disorders. The deformity consists of extreme dorsiflexion of the foot, and it can be distinguished from congenital vertical talus by its flexibility. If, after examination concern for vertical talus remains, radiographic evaluation can help with diagnosis. If left untreated, CCV may lead to symptomatic flatfoot later in life, leading to abnormal joint relationships and delayed or abnormal ambulation (**Fig. 8**).[25] In severe cases, the peroneal tendons may be involved; therefore these should be evaluated.[18]

Congenital Rigid Flatfoot

Congenital vertical talus
Congenital convex pes valgus, commonly known as vertical talus, is a rare flatfoot deformity. On physical examination, one will note equinus of the rearfoot and a rigid rocker bottom appearance. It is important to differentiate it from CCV by its rigid nature. Radiographs confirm the diagnosis, revealing the irreducible talonavicular joint and fixed equinus. Usually the deformity is detected at birth; otherwise the symptoms can begin at age of ambulation and can be quite devastating if left untreated.[26] In about half of the cases, it is associated with neuromuscular and genetic disorders; therefore it is important to rule these out during examination or with appropriate referrals.[27–29]

Tarsal coalitions
Congenital rigid flatfoot also can be caused by tarsal coalitions. The most commonly encountered coalitions are calcaneonavicular and talocalcaneal middle facet coalition, accounting for 90% of all coalitions.[30] Up to 50% of tarsal coalitions are found

Table 2
Comparing normal and abnormal radiographic values in pediatric pes planovalgus

Radiographic Angles	Normal		Pes Planus	
	AP	Lateral	AP	Lateral
TC	30°–40°	35°–40°	Increases	Increases
CIA		35°–40°		Decreases
TDA		30°		Increases
Talar-1st metatarsal		0°		Increases

Abbreviations: CIA, calcaneal inclination angle; TC, talocalcaneal; TDA, talar declination angle.

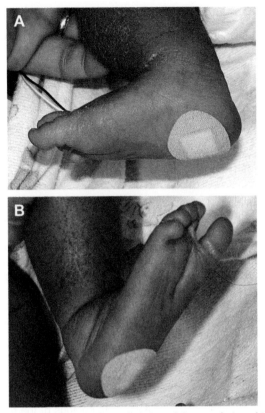

Fig. 5. Calcaneovalgus in a newborn. (*A*) Medial view. (*B*) Lateral view. (*Courtesy of* Neal M. Blitz, DPM, Bronx, New York.)

to be bilateral; therefore examination including radiographs should be done on both sides.[7] Age of onset depends on the coalition but generally will be found in older children, not infants.[31] Physical examination will reveal limitation of subtalar and midtarsal joint motion, deep pain or aching at the coalition site, or pain on palpation of the sinus

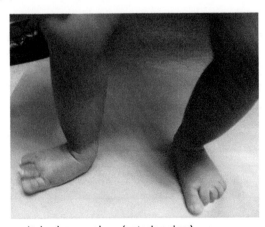

Fig. 6. Bilateral congenital calcaneovalgus (anterior view).

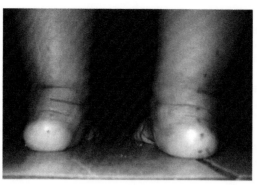

Fig. 7. Bilateral congenital calcaneovalgus (posterior view).

tarsi or sustentaculum tali or the entire rearfoot. The pain is reported to be aggravated by activity and relieved by rest. Peroneal spastic flatfoot also may be encountered; this could be caused by an underlying tarsal coalition or present as an isolated finding of undetermined etiology.[1,32]

Acquired Flexible Flatfoot

Most children presenting for evaluation of an acquired, flexible pes valgus deformity, with or without symptoms, will have abnormal, faulty biomechanical alignment of the lower extremity as the primary cause for an acquired, compensatory deformity of the foot. Most of these biomechanical etiologies originate in the superstructure; therefore, a comprehensive lower extremity examination should be performed. In starting prox-imally at the hips and ending distally, the examiner can identify all contributing factors to compensatory, closed-chain pronation of the subtalar joint. Identifying these super-structural influences presents an additional opportunity to recommend treatment of these proximal mal-alignments to realign them and to reduce their negative influences

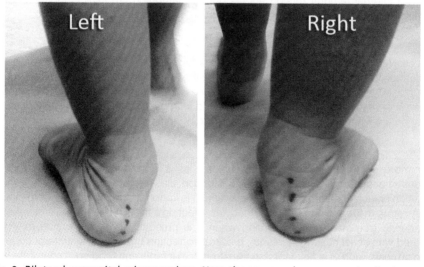

Fig. 8. Bilateral congenital calcaneovalgus. Note the severe calcaneus eversion in stance.

on the foot. The presence of cartilaginous, physeal bone and malleable soft tissue subjected to Davis' law allows the child's lower extremity to be guided and molded to a better-aligned position. Improved alignment of the child's superstructure will reduce negative forces on the foot and compensatory foot deformities over time.[11,33]

Comprehensive biomechanical assessment should include both weight-bearing and nonweight bearing examinations. It is easy to dismiss a foot as normal when only performing a nonweight bearing examination. Pathomechanical acquired pes valgus is a result of abnormal closed chain mechanics on weight bearing. It is only after the foot is loaded, closing the kinetic chain, that these pathomechanical influences of the superstructure on the subtalar joint and foot become evident. The subtalar joint functions normally to serve as the key to lock the foot in midstance phase of gait in preparation for heel lift and propulsion. Rigid lever function is required for normal propulsion. Superpedal and pedal influences contribute to prolonged pronation of the subtalar joint into midstance and beyond, leading to unlocking of the midtarsal joint and poor propulsive function.[34] These influences must be identified to properly and comprehensively evaluate a child for flexible, acquired pes valgus. Children with identifiable superstructural and infrastructural influences leading to compensatory out-of-phase pronation of the foot must be considered at risk for progressive deformity with potential to develop symptoms with increasing body weight and greater activity as they mature.[3–5,17,18,33–36]

BIOMECHANICAL ETIOLOGIES OF THE FLEXIBLE FLATFOOT
Hip and Femur

Excessive internal rotation of the hip accompanied by reduced external rotation in the transverse plane may place the neutral position of the child's hip more internally. This excessive internal rotation that can be caused by tight hip muscles is called internal femoral position and sometimes femoral anteversion. True femoral torsion, or osseous deformity or twist of the femur, can be differentiated using Ryder's test. If the medial condyle of the femur lies posterior to the lateral condyle with the greater trochanter maintained in the frontal plane, then internal femoral torsion (femoral antetorsion) is present. Femoral torsion angles of greater than 10° internal after maturity and retention of high internal femoral torsion angles during maturation are clinical indications of femoral antetorsion and should be noted when present.[13,14]

Knee

Excessive internal rotation of the knee joint (known as pseudotorsion or internal genicular position) produces an internal transverse plane influence on the subtalar joint in the closed kinetic chain. The infant with excessive rotation of the knee joint in the internal or medial direction may be diagnosed with pseudotorsion, and serial casting may be appropriate in the prewalking child to normalize the knee joint function.

Tibia

Far more common, and of greater concern as a significant etiology for flexible, acquired pes planovalgus, is internal tibial torsion, also referred to as internal malleolar position or lack of external malleolar position. It is important to remember not to externally rotate the femur and thus the condyles, creating a falsely external malleolar angle obscuring true internal tibial torsion when it is present.[15,16] Tibial torsion may be treated with serial casting in infants, bilateral correction orthosis, or unilateral correction orthosis such as a tibial torsion transformer in infants and toddlers to derotate the deformity.

Internal torsions of the femur and tibia and internally positioned soft tissue of the hip and knee joints place an internal rotatory force on the talus in the ankle mortise at the distal end of the tibia in the closed chain. Internal influences from the superstructure, often exacerbated by further internal rotations during the gait cycle, place an adductory or internal rotatory force on the talus. This facilitates combined closed-chain pronation of the subtalar joint that consists of talar adduction and plantarflexion with eversion of the calcaneus. This leads to pathomechanically induced flexible, acquired pes valgus in children. It is for this reason, among others, that positional deformities of the hip and knee joint and residual internal torsions of the femur and tibia should not be considered benign and without potential consequence. The inward angle of gait that may result from these conditions is often the presenting complaint in many of these children and only upon thorough weight-bearing examination of the foot is the compensatory foot pathology identified. Many of these children, although asymptomatic at the time of initial presentation, may be at considerable risk to develop symptoms with increasing body mass and greater sports participation. Prescribing foot orthoses in cases where these comorbidities have been identified may be prudent in helping to prevent the onset of symptoms over time and forestall other consequences known to be associated with long-standing pes planovalgus.

Among the most significant of potential compensations for equinus deformities of the lower extremity includes acquired, flexible pes valgus, notably with a breach or compensation at the midtarsal joint, often presenting with the classic rocker bottom, fully compensated equinovalgus foot type. Tightness of proximal muscles identified by the Thomas test may, through soft tissue connections to the distal gastrocnemius-solues complex, result in compensations at the foot level in joints with available sagittal plane range of motions such as the midtarsal joint.

Ankle

Tightness in either the gastrocnemius or solues muscles will increase the demand on the joints of the foot to provide the necessary dorsiflexion for gait. An acquired pes valgus deformity may result when equinus influences are present. These influences should be addressed through various options including heel raises, altered shoe heel heights, a stretching program, physical medicine, and rehabilitation referrals and, in severe, recalcitrant cases, surgical lengthening procedures or removal of bony blocks. Concurrent management of the compensatory, acquired pes valgus deformity should be considered to protect the growing foot from these destructive influences while the sagittal plane alignment of the child is improved.

Foot

When comparing RCSP and NCSP in a pediatric pes planovalgus deformity, improved morphology of the foot will be noted with reduction of double ankles from talar bulge and better hallux position in the frontal plane. In a forefoot varus, because the forefoot is inverted, the foot compensates by pronating at the subtalar joint to bring the midtarsal joint down, thus lowering the medial column to the floor. In children younger than 6 years, forefoot varus may resolve spontaneously with development. In a flexible forefoot valgus, the forefoot must invert, causing midtarsal joint supination to bring the forefoot to the ground, resulting in instability and hypermobility with eventual compensatory pronation.[17,19]

The foot functions as a unit based on the motion and resultant planal dominance of the subtalar, midtarsal, and ankle joints.[37] Planal dominance addresses each cardinal plane, determining the major plane in which the deformity is taking place, and the plane in which compensation is occurring, helping to determine the location of the subtalar joint axis. The low subtalar joint axis creates frontal plane compensation, resulting in calcaneal valgus. Frontal plane dominance can be appreciated on radiograph by a decreased first metatarsal declination angle and height of the sustentaculum, increased superposition of the lesser tarsus on lateral view, and a widening lesser tarsus on an anterior-posterior view.[38] On the other hand, a high subtalar joint axis creates transverse plan compensation, resulting in forefoot abduction and minimal calcaneal valgus.[34,35] This transverse planal dominance is demonstrated on an AP radiograph with an increased talocalcaneal angle, increased calcaneocuboid angle, decreased talonavicular congruency, and decreased forefoot-to-rearfoot adduction (**Fig. 9**). One would determine sagittal plane dominance on lateral radiographs with an increased talar declination angle, increased talocalcaneal angle, decreased calcaneal inclination angle, and naviculocuneiform breach (**Box 1**), (**Fig. 10**).[38]

ACQUIRED FLEXIBLE FLATFOOT SECONDARY TO TRAUMA

Two studies have reported on the occurrence of pes planus in children after rupture of the tibialis posterior tendon. One study reported on three young patients who developed unilateral pes planus after old undiagnosed lacerations of the posterior tibial tendon. These authors suggest that the presence of unilateral pes planus in a child should lead the clinician to examine the skin of the medial malleolar area for any evidence of prior injury.[8] The second study reported a single case of a tibialis posterior tendon rupture in a 10-year old child with ankle pain after a fall from a bicycle and twisting of her ankle. The ruptured tendon was discovered only 3 months after the injury when she presented with continued pain, limitation of activity, unilateral pes planovalgus, and inability to resupinate the rearfoot with a Hubscher maneuver.[9]

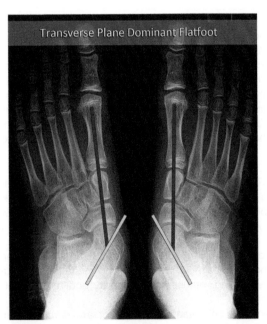

Fig. 9. Anterior-posterior radiograph demonstrating transverse planal dominance. Note the increased talocalcaneal angle, increased calcaneocuboid angle, decreased talonavicular congruency, and decreased forefoot-to-rearfoot adduction.

| **Box 1** |
| **List of deforming forces associated with acquired pes planovalgus** |
| *Sagittal Plane* |
| Equinus |
| Gastrosoleus |
| Hamstring |
| Iliopsoas |
| *Frontal Plane* |
| Genuvalgum |
| Forefoot varus |
| *Transverse Plane* |
| Femoral antetorsion |
| Internal femoral position |
| Internal tibial torsion |
| Morton's syndrome |
| Limb length discrepancy |

Rigid Acquired Flatfoot

Peroneal spastic flatfoot without coalition

Peroneal spastic flatfoot without coalition may occur for various reasons, including pain, trauma, infection, or arthritis of the hindfoot joints.[39,40] One study reports a case of a peroneal spastic flatfoot secondary to an osteochondral lesion of the talus. A 16-year-old boy presented with a unilateral peroneal spastic flatfoot that was found to have been caused by an ipsilateral talar osteochondral lesion detected on MRI.[39] This etiology should be considered in children with peroneal spastic flatfoot without evidence of tarsal coalition. Common peroneal nerve block has been advocated for peroneal spastic flatfoot in the presence or absence of tarsal coalition to allow better assessment of motion.[40]

Iatrogenic Rigid Flatfoot

Iatrogenic rigid flatfoot deformities, although uncommon, may result from overcorrected clubfoot, undercorrected vertical talus, failed flatfoot surgery, and end-stage

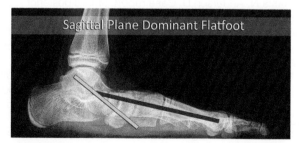

Fig. 10. Lateral radiograph demonstrating sagittal plane dominance. Note the increased talar declination angle, increased talocalcaneal angle, decreased calcaneal inclination angle, and naviculocuneiform breach.

trauma.[1] When dealing with these entities, it is imperative to obtain a detailed history of previous treatments and surgical interventions.

SUMMARY

The goal of clinical assessment is gaining a better understanding and appreciation for the deforming forces involved in pediatric pes planovalgus deformity. A thorough consistent clinical evaluation including a comprehensive history, physical examination, and supplemental imaging studies is critical in ascertaining the appropriate diagnosis of the various etiologies.

ACKNOWLEDGMENTS

The authors would like to take the time to thank their families and colleagues who have supported them with this paper, in particular Dr Neal Blitz, and Dr Danny Choung.

REFERENCES

1. Harris E, Vanore J, Thomas J, et al. Diagnosis and treatment of pediatric flatfoot: clinical practice guideline. J Foot Ankle Surg 2004;43(6):341–73.
2. Wenger DR, Leach J. Foot deformities in infants and children. Pediatr Clin North Am 1986;33:1411–27.
3. Lin C, Lai K, Kuan T, et al. Correlating factors and clinical significance of flexible flatfoot in preschool children. J Pediatr Orthop 2001;21(3):378–82.
4. Pheffer M, Kotz R, Ledl T, et al. Prevalence of flat foot in preschool-aged children. Pediatrics 2006;118:634–9.
5. Napolitano C, Walsh S, Mahoney L, et al. Risk factors that may adversely modify the natural history of the pediatric pronated foot. Clin Podiatr Med Surg 2000;17: 397–417.
6. Mickle K, Steele J, Munro B. Is the foot structure of preschool children moderated by gender? J Pediatr Orthop 2008;28(5):593–6.
7. Herring JA. The orthopaedic examination: clinical application. In: Herring JA, editor. Tachdjian's pediatric orthopaedics. 4th edition. Philadelphia: WB Saunders Company; 2008. p. 67–78, 1035–189.
8. Masterson E, Jagannathan S, Borton D, et al. Pes planus in childhood due to tibialis posterior tendon injuries, treatment by flexor hallucis longus tendon transfer. J Bone Joint Surg Br 1994;76-B(3):444–6.
9. Abosoa A, Tumia N, Anderson D. Case report: tibialis posterior tendon rupture in children. Injury 2003;34(11):866–7.
10. Villarroya MA, Esquivel JM, Tomás C, et al. Assessment of the medial longitudinal arch in children and adolescents with obesity: footprints and radiographic study. Eur J Pediatr 2009;168(5):559–67.
11. Volpe RG. Pediatric gait. In: Thomson P, Volpe RG, editors. Introduction to podopediatrics. 2nd edition. Edinburgh (UK): Churchill-Livingstone; 2001. p. 49–71.
12. Volpe RG. Alterations of gait in neuromuscular disease. Clin Podiatr Med Surg 1988;5(3):627–38.
13. Ryder CT, Crane L. Measuring femoral anteversion: the problem and a method. J Bone Joint Surg Am 1953;35-A:321–8.
14. Volpe RG. Evaluation and management of in-toe gait in the neurologically intact child. Clin Podiatr Med Surg 1997;14(1):57–85.

15. Cohen-Sobel E, Levitz SJ. Torsional development of the lower extremity. Implications for in-toe and out-toe treatment. J Am Podiatr Med Assoc 1991;81(7): 344–57.
16. Lang LM, Volpe RG. Measurement of tibial torsion. J Am Podiatr Med Assoc 1998;88(4):160–5.
17. Valmassy RL. Torsional and frontal plane conditions of the lower extremity. In: Thomson P, Volpe RG, editors. Introduction to podopediatrics. 2nd edition. Edinburgh (UK): Churchill-Livingstone; 2001. p. 231–55.
18. Connors JF, Wernick E, Lowy LJ, et al. Guidelines for evaluation and management of five common podopediatric conditions. J Am Podiatr Med Assoc 1998;88(5): 206–22.
19. Mahan KT, Flanigan KP. Pathologic pes valgus disorders. In: Banks AS, Downey MS, Martin DE, et al, editors. McGlamry's comprehensive textbook of foot and ankle surgery. Philadelphia: Lippincott Williams & Watkins; 2001. p. 799–899.
20. Harris RI, Beath T. Etiology of peroneal spastic flatfoot. J Bone Joint Surg 1948; 30:624–34.
21. Bresnahan PJ. Pediatric abnormalities of position. In: Christman RA, editor. Foot and ankle radiology. St Louis (MO): Churchhill Livingstone; 2003. p. 303–13.
22. Vaughan WH, Segal G. Tarsal coalition, with special reference to roentgenographic interpretation. Radiology 1953;60:855–63.
23. Pressman M. Biomechanics and surgical criteria for flexible pes valgus. J Am Podiatr Med Assoc 1982;77(1):7–13.
24. Kantali U, Yetkin H, Cila E. Footprint and radiographic analysis of the feet. J Pediatr Orthop 2001;21(2):225–8.
25. Cohen-Sobel E, Giorgini R, Velez Z. Combined technique for surgical correction of pediatric severe flexible flatfoot. J Foot Ankle Surg 1995;34(2):83–94.
26. Alaee F, Boehm S, Dobbs MB. A new approach to the treatment of congenital vertical talus. J Child Orthop 2007;1:165–74.
27. Jacobsen ST, Crawford AH. Congenital vertical talus. J Pediatr Orthop 1983;3: 306–10.
28. Dodge LD, Ashley RK, Gilbert RJ. Treatment of the congenital vertical talus: a retrospective review of 36 feet with long-term follow-up. Foot Ankle 1987;7: 326–32.
29. Hamanishi C. Congenital vertical talus: classification with 69 cases and new measurement system. J Pediatr Orthop 1984;4:318–26.
30. Stormont DM, Peterson HA. The relative incidence of tarsal coalition. Clin Orthop 1983;181:28–36.
31. Cowell HR, Elener V. Rigid painful flatfoot secondary to tarsal coalition. Clin Orthop 1983;177:54–60.
32. Downey MS. Tarsal coalition. In: Banks AS, Downey MS, Martin DE, et al, editors. McGlamry's comprehensive textbook of foot and ankle surgery. Philadelphia: Lippincott Williams & Watkins; 2001. p. 993–1031.
33. D'Amico JC. Developmental flatfoot. In: Thomson P, Volpe RG, editors. Introduction to podopediatrics. 2nd edition. Edinburgh (UK): Churchill-Livingstone; 2001. p. 257–76.
34. Root ML, Orien WP, Weed JH. In: Normal and abnormal function of the foot: clinical biomechanics, vol. 2. Los Angeles (CA): Clinical Biomechanics Corporation; 1977. p. 75–93.
35. Manter JT. Movements of the subtalar and transverse tarsal joints. Anat Rec 1941; 80:397.

36. Green DR, Whitney A, Walters P. Subtalar joint motion: a simplified view. J Am Podiatry Assoc 1979;69:83.
37. Green DR, Carol A. Planal dominance. J Am Podiatry Assoc 1984;74(2):98--103.
38. Labovitz JM. The algorithmic approach to pediatric flexible pes planovalgus. Clin Podiatr Med Surg 2006;23:57–76.
39. Blair J, Perdios A, Reilly C. Peroneal spastic flatfoot caused by osteochondral lesion: a case report. Foot Ankle Int 2007;28(6):724–6.
40. Lowy LJ. Pediatric peroneal spastic flatfoot in the absence of coalition: a suggested protocol. J Am Podiatr Med Assoc 1998;88:181–91.
41. Valmassay RL. Biomechanical examination of the child. In: Valmassay RL, editor. Clinical biomechanics of the lower extremity. St Louis (MO): Mosby; 1996. p. 244–77.

Flexible Pediatric and Adolescent Pes Planovalgus: Conservative and Surgical Treatment Options

Neal M. Blitz, DPM, FACFAS[a],*, Robert J. Stabile, DPM, AACFAS[b],
Renato J. Giorgini, DPM[c], Lawrence A. DiDomenico, DPM[d,e]

KEYWORDS

• Flexible flatfoot • Pes planovalgus • Equinus

Symptomatic flexible pediatric pes planovalgus is a common problem encountered in the foot and ankle practice. There is a wide range of clinical presentations, both objectively and subjectively. Structurally, the feet may be mildly flat to severely flat, and may occur in a single plane or multiple planes. In this patient population, growth plates are typically open (skeletally immature) or near closure, which directly affects the treatment recommendations and pathways. The treatment goals are directed first at resolution of pain, and second at the realignment of the foot. Conservative management should be attempted before surgical intervention. Surgical reconstruction and the procedure selection are based on the physical examination, radiographs (standing), planal dominance, and resultant biomechanical compensations.[1] This article provides an overview of the common treatment pathways that highlight methods to structurally realign the pediatric and adolescent flatfoot.

[a] Department of Orthopaedic Surgery, Bronx-Lebanon Hospital Center, 1650 Selwyn Avenue, Bronx, NY 10457, USA
[b] Division of Podiatry, Department of Surgery, Nassau University Medical Center, 2201 Hempstead Turnpike, East Meadow, NY 11554, USA
[c] Division of Podiatry, Good Samaritan Hospital Medical Center, 1000 Montauk Highway, West Islip, NY 11795, USA
[d] Ohio College of Podiatric Medicine, 6000 Rockside Woods Boulevard Independence, OH 44131, USA
[e] Section of Podiatric Medicine and Surgery, St Elizabeth Hospital, 1044 Belmont Avenue, Youngstown, OH 44504-1096, USA
* Corresponding author.
E-mail address: nealblitz@yahoo.com (N.M. Blitz).

Clin Podiatr Med Surg 27 (2010) 59–77
doi:10.1016/j.cpm.2009.09.001
0891-8422/09/$ – see front matter © 2010 Elsevier Inc. All rights reserved.

CONSERVATIVE MANAGEMENT

The conservative management of flexible flatfoot begins with education of the patient and the parents. Education should consist of the biomechanical findings that support the diagnosis of a flatfoot and the purpose of corrective devices if used. Different severities of deformity are present ranging from mild to the very severe symptomatic flatfoot. Some cases may be so mild that no treatment is indicated at the time; normal development and strengthening of the foot may be all the treatment indicated. Obtaining a family history, particularly of the parents and the patient's siblings about any similar problems, may be insightful about the genetic structure of the child's foot and provide a realm of familiarity to the parents concerning treatment for their child's condition.

Promoting and discussing proper supportive shoe gear is an important first-line treatment in the flexible flatfoot. Typically, an enclosed sneaker offers structural support to the skeletally immature foot. The sneaker should comfortably support an orthotic device if that is to be the next line of treatment. The shoe should have a firm sole to prevent the orthosis from compressing the medial side of the shoe.[2] High-top sneakers may be indicated if a large amount of instability is present within the ankle and subtalar joints. Certain types of shoes such as sandals and moccasin styles should be discouraged because they may fail to provide the structural support that the skeletally immature patient needs.

Passive stretching of the tendo-Achilles complex can be done if an equinus deformity exists, and the stretching should be part of the conservative approach to flexible flatfoot. Equinus can be a strong deforming force in the sagittal plane and also influences the frontal and transverse plane position. Statically and dynamically, an equinus contracture can result in the breakdown of the midfoot, clinically seen as flattening of the arch and abduction of the midfoot. One may visualize equinus dynamically as an early heel-off in gait. Multiple exercises for stretching the Achilles tendon can be easily taught to the patient. Active strengthening exercises do not provide any benefit to an equinus condition unless a muscle weakness is noted.

Nonsteroidal anti-inflammatory drugs may be used if symptoms of inflammation are present. Medial column collapse and strain may present as an inflammatory process and warrant the use of anti-inflammatory medications in conjunction with resting and icing to alleviate the symptoms. Apophysitis is common in the skeletally immature patient and requires similar treatment.

Orthotic therapy in the pediatric flexible flatfoot helps restore structure and support to the medial column. The purpose of a functional orthosis is to control the amount of pronation across the subtalar joint, thereby restoring the support and alignment to the talocalcaneal joint. Either an increase in the supination moment or a decrease in the pronation moment will achieve the desired result on weight bearing.[2] According to Valmassy,[3] a functional orthosis device is only appropriate for use in a pediatric patient after a heel-to-toe gait has begun. According to Jay and colleagues,[4] a pediatric orthotic device should attempt to accommodate the intrinsic and extrinsic structural deformities, provide rigidity for control but accommodate the natural foot shape, create postural alignment of the foot to the leg, and finally contain materials that enhance the patient-orthoses interface. As a first-line orthotic treatment, the dynamic stabilizing innersole system serves to control hyperpronation in young children via stabilization of the medial and lateral columns and to control calcaneal eversion through a deep heel seat. This device is typically used in the first few years after ambulation has begun.[4] The University of California at Berkeley Laboratory (UCBL) orthotic device is another example of a device that can control the flexible flatfoot deformity demonstrating hyperpronation and to be used early in the child's life. The advantage of the UCBL orthotic device is its high medial and lateral flanges to provide control of the rearfoot and midfoot complexes, especially when increased transverse plane deformity is seen. Other foot orthoses types that have been used in the pediatric population are Whitman-Roberts orthoses, heel stabilizers, and Schaffer type orthoses.[4]

Compliance can become an issue with these devices and may require thorough explanation and education to the parents. A discussion of how the orthotics function to help support and provide realignment to the foot may be beneficial in helping the parents understand why such a treatment is necessary. In addition, visual aids, such as a skeleton foot model placed over an actual orthotic device, can demonstrate the ability of the device to capture the foot and prevent arch collapse. It allows the patient and parents to visualize the purpose of the prescribed device.

For the more severe flatfooted deformity or the ligamentous laxed patient, in whom ankle instability, posterior tibial tendon symptoms, or early arthrosis has developed, an ankle-foot orthosis (AFO) or a more proximal device can be more appropriate. The adolescent, skeletally mature patient may benefit somewhat from these types of orthoses or as a last line of nonsurgical treatment. The goal of these devices is to facilitate the transmission of deforming forces onto external materials, and to assist normal ground reactive forces through corrected functional anatomy and alignment.[5] In case of equinus, in which there is restriction of ankle joint range of motion, specific devices such as rocker bottom shoe soles, torque absorbing AFOs, and proximal weight-bearing AFOs can be used.

SURGICAL TREATMENT

Surgical intervention for the flexible pediatric flatfoot is typically reserved for symptomatic feet that have not responded to conservative measures. The goals of surgery are simple: pain reduction or resolution and realignment of the foot. Although attaining these goals may be difficult because there are such a wide variety of clinical presentations ranging from mild flatfeet to severe flatfeet with a multitude of planal dominance contributions, that surgical realignment may be challenging. A variety of surgical methods have been described to correct the flexible pediatric flatfoot, and they are categorized in 3 types: (1) reconstructive osteotomies (extra-articular), (2) arthroereisis, and/or (3) arthrodesis.[6,7] Less commonly considered as a distinct category are the medial column soft tissue procedures (**Box 1**).

Flatfoot procedure selection often involves a combination of these types of procedures and it is critical to understand the pathomechanics and planal dominance of each individual foot as a separate entity when considering surgical intervention and developing a strategic surgical plan. Although many of the surgical procedures may be performed individually, often reconstructions involve a combination of soft tissue and osseous procedures (osteotomies and/or fusions) to achieve correction. In addition to the level and degree of deformity, surgeons must also consider age and skeletal maturity.

SURGICAL MANAGEMENT OF EQUINUS

Equinus correction is almost universally performed along with a pediatric flatfoot correction. The contribution of gastrocnemius, soleus, and/or both the muscle groups to equinus dictates the surgical management. The Silfverskiold test is necessary to determine the location of contracture, and is covered elsewhere in this issue. Isolated gastrocnemius contracture may be resolved with a gastrocnemius recession and multiple techniques may be used.[8] A Strayer recession involves completely transecting the gastrocnemius aponeurosis, thus eliminating gastrocnemius contribution,[9,10] although surgical reattachment, or scaring down of this aponeurosis, may provide

---

Box 1
Surgical treatment categories for flexible flatfoot

Arthroereisis

    Subtalar

Soft tissue medial column procedures

    Kidner procedure

    Young tenosuspension

    Modified Kidner-Cobb

Osteotomies

    Medial column

        Cotton medial cuneiform

    Rearfoot

        Medializing calcaneal osteotomy

        Evans calcaneal osteotomy

        Double calcaneal osteotomy

Arthrodesis

    Medial column

        Lapidus

        Hoke

        Miller

    Rearfoot

        Isolated talonavicular joint

        Isolated subtalar joint

        Isolated calcaneocuboid joint and/or distraction

        Double rearfoot fusion

        Triple arthrodesis

---

some return of gastrocnemius function in a lengthened state. Gastrocnemius equinus may also be managed by lengthening only the muscular bound gastrocnemius aponeurosis (gastrocnemius intramuscular aponeurotic recession or Baumann), which theoretically only weakens the gastrocnemius pull while preserving the natural anatomic insertional attachment of gastrocnemius onto soleus.[11–14] When concomitant soleus equinus exists, aponeurotic lengthening of soleus may also be performed. Endoscopic gastrocnemius recession has also been used.[15] The Vulpius procedure and Baker tongue-in-groove recession are other methods to manage gastrosoleal equinus above the Achilles tendon (**Fig. 1**).[8,16,17] Alternatively, surgeons may perform a tendo-Achilles lengthening through an open or percutaneous technique.

Arthroereisis

Subtalar arthroereisis describes a procedure where a spacer is placed into the sinus tarsi, restricting pronation.[6] Pronatory forces can be reduced by limiting the contact of the lateral talar process against the calcaneal sinus tarsi floor, therefore maintaining a more neutral position of the talocalcaneal joint. It is a means of reducing joint motion

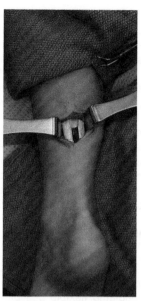

Fig. 1. Tongue-in-groove gastrocnemius recession for gastrosoleus equinus in pediatric patient.

without sacrificing total loss of motion (ie, arthrodesis) to provide stability to the rearfoot. It should be noted that arthroereisis is used as an adjunctive procedure, which can be powerful in correcting frontal plane deformity.

Historically, arthroereisis involved extra-articular bony blocks.[18–20] Nowadays, most arthroereisis procedures involve implants (removable, if necessary) that are less invasive and do not require cutting, drilling, or direct implantation into the calcaneus. Several products currently exist on the market for this procedure, and differences in the design of these implants are not discussed in this article, but the purpose of the implant is to be "well-seated" within the sinus tarsi, thus preventing collapse of this space (ie, pronation).

A distinct advantage of the arthroereisis procedure in the pediatric population is that the implant provides structural realignment of the rearfoot complex during skeletal growth, which may become a permanent correction as the child reaches and surpasses skeletal maturity. As such, the implant may be removed as the child skeletally matures. According to Giannini,[21] surgery performed during growth provides an optimal and lasting correction of the deformity, restoring the talocalcaneal alignment with remodeling of the subtalar joint.

More contemporary are the bioabsorbable implants that obviously do not require removal. However, potential limitations include foreign body reaction and surgical challenges when placing the radio-translucent implant. The bioabsorbable and metallic implants have been reported to occasionally cause symptoms requiring explantation of the device, however these reports occurred in adults.[22,23] It is possible that pediatric patients may better tolerate a sinus tarsi implant because skeletal immaturity may adapt to a changing environment.

Proper sizing and placement of the implant, whether it is absorbable or metallic, is crucial to the success of the arthroereisis procedure. Too large an implant may result in lateral symptoms and too small may result in under correction.[22] Assessment of the range of motion should be performed on the talocalcaneal joint intraoperatively after insertion of the trial implants to achieve a neutral position. Pronation of the subtalar joint should be restricted but not eliminated. Intraoperative fluoroscopy to visualize the transverse position of the implant within the sinus tarsi is also used. The leading (medial) edge of the implant should be placed at the bisection of the talus.

Arthroereisis may be used in isolation for flexible flatfoot repair or in combination with other reconstructive flatfoot procedures, such as soft tissue procedures of the medial column, osteotomies, and/or fusions. The individuality of these procedures are discussed later, but the theoretical concept is that the "pronation blockade" by arthroereisis helps support the subacute postsurgical healing of medial column procedures (soft tissue and/or osseous) by preventing collapse from premature weight bearing. In addition, while the subtalar arthroereisis corrects the rearfoot malalignment, it may uncover a concomitant forefoot varus once the rearfoot is aligned (**Fig. 2**) and surgeons may want to consider combining the reconstruction with a medial column procedure that brings the medial column into alignment.

SOFT TISSUE MEDIAL COLUMN RECONSTRUCTIONS
The Kidner Procedure

The Kidner procedure is best known for its place in removal of a symptomatic accessory navicular (os tibiale externum) or hypertrophic navicular, which may often be a pathologic component of pediatric flexible pes planovalgus.[24] The presence of this accessory bone has been implicated in transmitting a functional disadvantage to the posterior tibialis tendon (the most significant inverter of the foot). One study reported that the presence of an accessory navicular plays no role in the development of a flatfoot.[25] An accessory navicular may be a pain producer if enlarged and/or synchondrotic with the navicular. Advanced imaging with computed tomography (CT) and/or magnetic resonance imaging (MRI) may be invaluable in making this distinction, whereas bone scan has not been shown to be useful.[26] The main role of

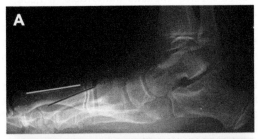

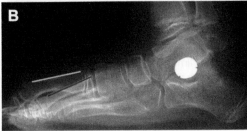

Fig. 2. Preoperative (A) and postoperative (B) lateral weight-bearing radiographs of subtalar arthroereisis in skeletally immature patient. The forefoot varus is evident after the arthroereisis realigns the rearfoot. Note the elevation of the first ray (dorsal cortex of the first metatarsal joint, *green line*) compared with the second metatarsal joint (dorsal cortex of the second metatarsal, *purple line*). A flexible forefoot varus should correct over time.

the Kidner procedure (a soft tissue medial column procedure) is to restore the mechanical advantage of the posterior tibial tendon. Other procedures that balance and/or structurally realign the foot may be required, especially procedures involving the rearfoot and/or lateral column (**Fig. 3**).

Bennett and colleagues[27] reported their retrospective review of 50 consecutive patients (75 feet) with symptomatic accessory navicular or prominent navicular tuberosity who underwent simple excision without alteration of the tibialis posterior course. Good or excellent results were reported by 90% of the patients. Koop and Marcus[28] retrospectively reviewed the Kidner procedure on 13 consecutive patients (14 feet) for simple resection of symptomatic accessory navicular bones, in a slightly older patient population (mean age 28.2 years), demonstrating an average postoperative American Orthopaedic Foot and Ankle Society (AOFAS) score of 94.5. Tan and colleagues[29] compared simple ossicle resection versus the Kidner procedure in 18 patients, over an average follow-up time of 3.1 years, and they demonstrated that both procedures alleviated symptoms in 15 of the 18 patients. Prichasuk and Sinphurmsukskul,[30] in their review of 28 patients, identified that the isolated Kidner procedure itself did not significantly restore the medial longitudinal arch,. These studies support the contention that the main purpose of the Kidner procedure is to manage the protuberance of the navicular and/or accessory ossicle and that it should not be considered as a major reconstructive procedure to restore the medial longitudinal arch when performed in isolation.

The surgical approach involves a medially based incision directly over the hypertrophic navicular tuberosity and/or os tibialis externum. Esthetically, surgeons should consider a concave incision (keeping in mind the relaxed skin tension lines) because this orientation gives the appearance of an arch when healed, which is advantageous when correcting a flatfoot deformity. The posterior tibialis is detached from the accessory navicular maintaining as much length of the tendon as possible. Once the ossicle is removed, any enlargement or prominence of the navicular tuberosity is also removed. The posterior tibialis tendon may be advanced on the navicular tuberosity, and placed inferiorly to restore its native attachment. Reattachment is most routinely performed with bone anchors, placing the foot in an inverted and plantar flexed position. Postoperative course involves non–weight bearing until the tenodesis has healed, a process that may take 6 to 8 weeks.

Modified Kidner-Cobb

The modified Kidner-Cobb procedure is a modification of the Kidner procedure, where a section of tibialis anterior is used to reinforce the insertion of the posterior tibial repair (**Fig. 4**).[31–34] Because the section of the tibialis anterior that is transferred is no longer connected to the pulling action of the tibialis anterior, the adjunctive nature of this procedure is merely to support other medial column soft tissue work. In 2003, Viegas[35] reviewed 17 consecutive pediatric patients (34 feet), over a 5-year period, who underwent reconstruction of flexible pediatric pes planus using a medial split tibialis anterior tendon in conjunction with a Kidner, Evans, and tendo-Achilles lengthening. Radiographic measurements improved statistically with the aforementioned reconstruction.

It is the authors' opinion that this modification be considered when (1) significant degeneration of the posterior tibialis tendon has occurred, (2) there is difficulty reattaching the posterior tibial tendon after a large os tibiale externum is removed and/or a large navicular tuberosity is resected, and (3) it is necessary for a spring ligament support.

Young Tibialis Anterior Tenosuspension

This soft tissue procedure, first described in 1939, involves inferior transpositioning of the tibialis anterior tendon through a slit or a hole in the navicular tuberosity, while

66

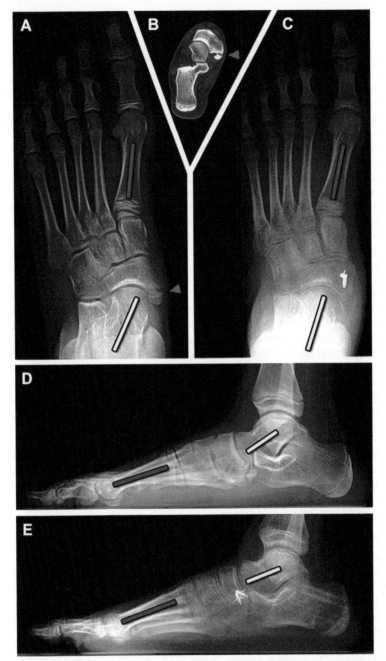

Fig. 3. 12-year-old skeletally immature girl with a symptomatic painful pes planovalgus and accessory navicular. Flatfoot reconstruction involved Kidner procedure with bone anchors and a medializing calcaneal osteotomy. (*A, D*) Preoperative weight-bearing radiographs. (*B*) Preoperative CT scan illustrates the synchondrosis (*red arrowhead*) between the accessory bone and the navicular. A fragmented interface suggests that the union may be interrupted. (*C, E*) Postoperative weight-bearing radiographs. In addition to excising the accessory bone, the enlarged navicular was also resected. The calcaneal osteotomy was fixated with smooth Steinmann pins (removed) as the calcaneal apophysis was open at the time of surgery. Realignment of this foot is evident as the talo-first metatarsal angle is restored in the transverse and the sagittal planes (*yellow* and *blue lines*). Patient is pain free.

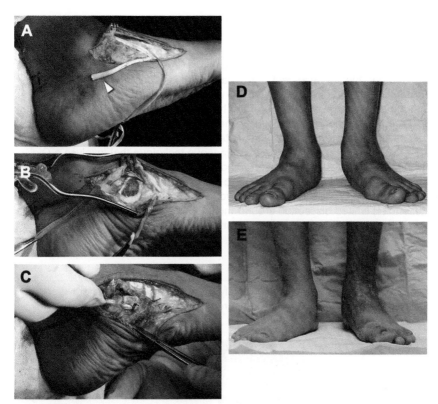

Fig. 4. Intraoperative series demonstrating the modified Kidner-Cobb technique. (*A*) The inferior portion of tibialis anterior is split. Proximally, the inferior half of the tendon is transected, and distally the attachment remains intact. (*B*) An enlarged navicular tuberosity is resected exposing cancellous bone. (*C*) Kidner procedure is performed (reattachment of the tibilais posterior to the navicular tuberosity) and reinforced with the split tibialis anterior tendon. (*D*) Clinical images before left foot reconstruction involving percutaneous tendo-Achilles lengthening, modified Kidner-Cobb, and subtalar joint arthroereisis. (*E*) Postoperative clinical image demonstrating improved medial arch height.

keeping its native attachment onto the first metatarsocuneiform joint intact.[36] This procedure has fallen out of favor with more advanced techniques available, but nonetheless, surgeons may see indications for its use on a case-by-case basis. In 1995, Cohen-Sobel and colleagues[37] performed the modified Young tenosuspension in conjunction with Evans calcaneal osteotomy and tendo-Achilles lengthening in 10 patients (12 feet) for severe flatfeet. In 1997, Dragonetti and colleagues[38] reported their retrospective results by comparing subtalar arthroereisis and tendo-Achilles lengthening with or without Young tenosuspension in 2 series of 15 feet. With regard to outcomes, the only statistically significant difference between the groups was the reduction of forefoot supination in the group that underwent Young tenosuspension.[38]

RECONSTRUCTION INVOLVING OSTEOTOMIES
Medializing Calcaneal Osteotomy

The medial calcaneal osteotomy is a common procedure in flatfoot reconstruction.[39,40] It is most useful when frontal plane deformity of the posterior calcaneal tuberosity exists (valgus of the heel). The procedure structurally realigns the calcaneus beneath the leg, which restores the biomechanical advantage of the Achilles tendon as a rearfoot inverter. Several techniques have been described.[41,42] Classically, the procedure involves an oblique lateral incision over the tuber, such that the sural nerve is avoided and the lateral aspect of the calcaneus is accessed at a level posterior to the subtalar joint and distal to the insertions of the Achilles tendon and plantar fascia. A through and through osteotomy of the heel allows the posterior tuber to be transposed medially. Although an obliquely linear osteotomy seems to be most popular, surgeons have also described other osteotomy orientations, such as a calcaneal scarf.[43] More contemporary is the percutaneous technique that involves a Gigli saw (**Fig. 5**).[44] The advantages of this method include (1) avoidance of the sural nerve, thus lessening the chance for iatrogenic sural nerve complications, (2) potentially less soft tissue complications (such as wound dehiscence), (3) cosmetically considerate, and (4) limited dissection around the lateral rearfoot allowing for less stress of the soft tissue for other concomitant nearby procedures to be performed within the same surgical setting.

Evans Calcaneal Osteotomy

Evans calcaneal osteotomy is used mainly for transverse plane flatfoot deformity by lengthening the lateral column.[45] The procedure is popular because it allows for

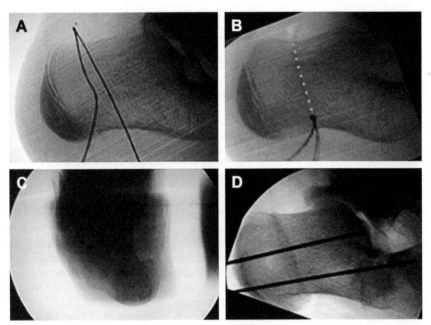

Fig. 5. Intraoperative fluoroscopic series demonstrating the technique for percutaneous calcaneal displacement osteotomy. (*A*) Gigli saw placement verified before performing the osteotomy. The osteotomy should be within the body of the calceaneal tuber, anterior to Achilles tendon insertion (and/or physis), and posterior to the subtalar joint. (*B*) The osteotomy is performed from superior to inferior direction. Here the Gigli saw is just about to penetrate the inferior calcaneal cortex for a through and through osteotomy. (*C*) Axial view demonstrating medial displacement of posterior fragment of tuber. (*D*) Fixation with 2 smooth K wires (or Steinmann pins), when the physis is open.

extra-articular correction of flatfoot deformity, which is especially desirable in the adolescent patient (**Fig. 6**). Traditionally, lengthening is achieved by inserting a bone graft into the anterior aspect of the calcaneus through a transverse osteotomy. Surgeons have varied the orientation of the osteotomy, the graft material (autograft, allograft, and synthetic), the absence and/or presence of a medial hinge, and the fixation constructs.[46,47] The amount of lengthening varies and is determined by the clinical scenario (ie, degree of deformity), and it is often an intraoperative decision as the surgeon can dial-in the amount of lengthening. Graft sizes of 5 to 15 mm have been used. Complications of the Evans procedure include delayed union, nonunion, malunion, subluxation of the calcaneocuboid joint, and persistent lateral column pain. The cause of lateral column pain may be related to jamming of the calcaneocuboid joint as contact characteristic studies after Evans procedure demonstrated increased pressure and altered contact patterns.[48,49] A cadaveric study by DiNucci and colleagues[50] measured strain on the long plantar ligament with sequentially increasing graft size with Evans procedure. They concluded that grafts more than 6 mm have no additional corrective capacity without compromising the long plantar ligament. Either larger graft size or loss of the long plantar ligament could compromise the intrinsic stability of the lateral column of the foot.[50] Another cadaveric study performed by Tien and colleagues[51] suggested that lateral column lengthening caused increased lateral forefoot plantar pressure, which was more pronounced during calcaneocuboid distraction arthrodesis than the Evans procedure. A more contemporary approach at lengthening is callus distraction with external fixation,[52] which allows for gradual lengthening (both the bone and soft tissue) with time, but it is criticized for the need for an external fixator.

Mosca[53] performed flatfoot reconstructions (or skew foot reconstructions) in 20 patients with Evans calcaneal osteotomy for symptomatic severe flatfoot. In 5 patients with skew foot, a Cotton medial cuneiform osteotomy was also performed. Follow-up was from approximately 5 to 16 years from the index operation. Satisfactory clinical

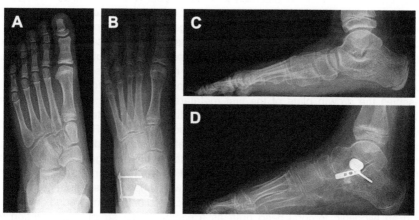

Fig. 6. Evans calcaneal osteotomy combined with subtalar arthroesis in an 11-year-old boy with flexible pes planus. (*A, C*) Preoperative weight-bearing images demonstrate transverse plane and sagittal plane deformity at the talonavicular joint. Dorsilateral peritalar subluxation and calcaneal cuboid abduction is present. (*B, D*) Postoperative images. Comparison of the anteroposterior views illustrate how the Evans osteotomy is capable of correcting the cuboid abduction. The lateral postoperative image is non–weight bearing. (*Courtesy of Dan Choung, DPM, San Rafael, CA.*)

and radiographic correction was achieved in all but 2 patients. He concluded that the aforementioned extra-articular reconstruction resolved the flatfoot-associated symptoms and avoided the need for arthrodeses procedures.[53] Davitt and colleagues[54] performed distal calcaneal lengthenings in children and adolescents (11 feet, 9 patients) and demonstrated improved radiographic values (talonavicular coverage angle and talo-first metatarsal angle, in a mean follow-up of 11.1 months). Ten of the 11 feet had excellent or good postoperative AOFAS scores.

Double Calcaneal Osteotomy (Medializing Calcaneal Osteotomy and Evans Calcaneal Osteotomy)

Surgeons have combined the benefits of the transverse plane correction achieved with Evans osteotomy and the frontal plane correction achieved with the medializing calcaneal osteotomy of the tuber, by performing a double calcaneal osteotomy for adolescent and adult flatfoot.[55] Catanzariti and colleagues[42] used the procedure in 8 patients with either adolescent flatfoot or adult late stage II posterior tibial tendon dysfunction. Moseir-LaClair and colleagues[56] performed 28 adult flatfoot reconstructions using a double calcaneal osteotomy combined with flexor tendon transfer and tendo-Achilles lengthening. The mean postoperative ankle-hindfoot AOFAS score was 90 with a mean follow-up of 5 years.[56]

A major advantage of the double calcaneal osteotomy in adolescent patients is that multiple planes of deformity can be corrected with preservation of the growth plates. In addition, the procedure is a joint sparing procedure. When performing the double calcaneal osteotomy, surgeons must be considerate of the incisional approach because accessing the anterior and posterior aspect of the calcaneus through a lateral approach may strain the soft tissue and result in dehiscence. A minimally invasive approach to the medializing calcaneal osteotomy component of the double calcaneal osteotomy may be beneficial.

Cotton Medial Cuneiform Osteotomy

The Cotton medial cuneiform osteotomy[57] is a procedure known for its use in pediatric and adolescent flexible flatfoot, and it is used for medial column collapse. The procedure calls for the insertion of an opening wedge bone graft (apex plantar) into the midsubstance of the medial cuneiform for the main purpose of sagittal plane correction of the collapsed medial column, although mild transverse plane correction may also be achieved. The procedure seems to be most advantageous in children and the adolescent population with flexible pes planovalgus deformities because it preserves the growth plate of the first metatarsal base in the skeletally immature patient, when medial column arthrodesis may otherwise be contraindicated.

Use of medial cuneiform osteotomies date back to 1908, when Riedel used a closing wedge osteotomy for hallux abducto valgus deformities to address the "atavistic" cuneiform.[58,59] In 1910, Young[60] reported on the opening wedge osteotomy for the correction of hallux abducto valgus, although Fowler[61] popularized the osteotomy for correction of forefoot adduction associated with a cavovarus deformity. In 1935, Cotton[57] (after whom the procedure is named) reported on opening wedge osteotomy using an allogenic femoral head graft as a sagittal plane structural correction for a depressed medial column in pes planus.

The Cotton osteotomy is rarely used as an isolated procedure in flatfoot reconstructions, however (**Fig. 7**) it is often combined with procedures that realign the rearfoot. It is well known that a compensatory forefoot varus exists in flexible flatfoot deformities, which becomes accentuated with correction of the rearfoot. The Cotton osteotomy corrects this deformity by plantar flexing the medial column, establishing an

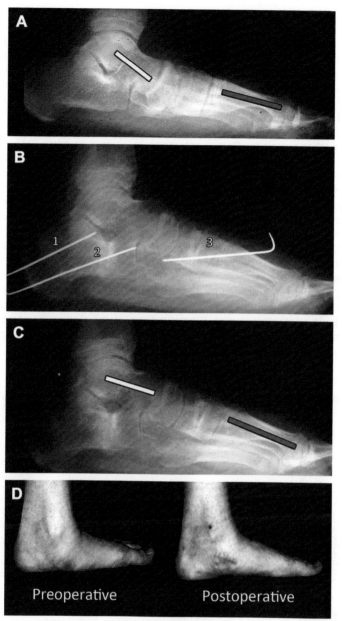

Fig. 7. Flatfoot reconstruction involved the following procedures: endoscopic gastrocnemius recession, double calcaneal osteotomy, Cotton osteotomy, and first metatarsal base osteotomy. (*A*) Preoperative weight-bearing lateral radiograph demonstrating the disruption of the talo-first metatarsal alignment (*yellow* and *blue lines*) with naviculocuneiform sag. Note the open physis demonstrating skeletal immaturity. (*B*) Postoperative lateral radiograph demonstrating the extra-articular osteotomies and fixation placement: (1) medial calcaneal displacement osteotomy, (2) Evans calcaneal osteotomy, and (3) Cotton medial cuneiform osteotomy and first metatarsal base osteotomy. (*C*) Postoperative weight-bearing radiographs demonstrating healing of all osteotomies and restoration of proper talo-first metatarsal alignment (*yellow* and *blue lines*). (*D*) Clinical preoperative and postoperative images of the aforementioned procedures demonstrating obvious visual improvement of the medial longitudinal arch.

immediate appropriate forefoot to rearfoot relationship.[57] The advantages of this technique (compared with first tarsometatarsal arthrodesis) include predictable union, preservation of first ray mobility, preservation of the open growth plate, and the ability to easily vary the amount of correction. However, the procedure should only be performed after ossification of the medial cuneiform (typically in children more than 6 years of age). Napiontek[62] has performed the Cotton procedure in 25 children less than 4 years of age.

The surgical approach for Cotton osteotomy involves a dorsomedial incision over the medial cuneiform (**Fig. 8**). The tibialis anterior and extensor hallucis longus are avoided. It is best to visualize the dorsal and medial aspects of the medial cuneiform, and use intraoperative fluoroscopy to identify the center of the cuneiform, as the optimal site for the osteotomy. A vertical osteotomy is made, all the way through the plantar cortex and a laminar spreader is used to open the medial cuneiform in the desired plane or planes to make the appropriate anatomic correction. A wedge-shaped tricortical cancellous graft is inserted to maintain the aforementioned desired anatomic correction. The goal is to bring the medial column down, limit the dorsal sagittal plane motion and, in some cases, to adjunctively correct transverse plane pathology. Because the procedure is most often used in the pediatric population with open growth plates, the bone graft is stabilized with smooth wires, although surgeons have used staples also. Complications of the Cotton procedure include tibialis anterior tendon injury, graft extrusion, irritation to the surrounding soft tissues, malalignment, nonunion, and delayed union.

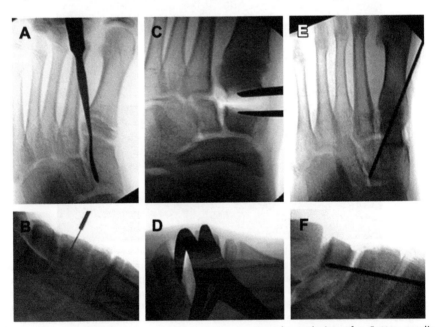

Fig. 8. Intraoperative fluoroscopic series demonstrating the technique for Cotton medial cuneiform osteotomy. (A, B) The position of the osteotomy should be verified before making the medial cuneiform. A freer elevator may be used to define the interval between the medial cuneiform and intermediate cuneiform. (C, D) A lamina spreader is used to create a wedge within the medial cuneiform with the base dorsal and apex plantar. (E, F) After the bone graft is placed fixation should be performed; in this case a smooth K wire was used.

RECONSTRUCTION INVOLVING ARTHRODESIS
Medial Column Arthrodesis (Lapidus ± Navicular Cuneiform)

Medial column arthrodesis procedures are considered when the flexible flatfoot is associated with skeletal maturity or when the growth plates are near closed (**Figs. 9** and **10**). The procedures are indicated for medial column instability that results in collapse. The radiographic location of the collapse determines the level/location of fusion. Isolated fusions of the first tarsometatarsal joint (Lapidus)[63] or the navicular cuneiform joint (Hoke)[64] have been used. The first tarsometatarsal and navicular cuneiform joint may be concomitantly fused, often referred to as the Miller procedure.[65]

Dockery[66] advocated medial column fusion to correct medial column instability as an adjunctive procedure in the surgical treatment of symptomatic juvenile flexible flatfoot. el-Tayeby[7] combined medial column fusion (naviculocuneiform joint) along with Evans, tendo-Achilles lengthening, and plantar rerouting of the tibialis anterior tendon in 11 patients (19 feet) with an average age of 10.7 years. Naviculocuneiform fixation was achieved with 2 crossing Kirschner wires (K wires) and nonunion occurred in 2 cases. Statistically significant improvement in radiographic alignment was achieved with this technique.[7]

Rearfoot Arthrodesis

The use of rearfoot arthrodesis for the treatment of symptomatic flexible juvenile flatfoot is limited. Selective arthrodeses or triple arthrodesis may be performed in the case of severe painful deformity, although selective arthrodeses should be strongly considered over triple arthrodesis. In general, rearfoot fusion of essential joints is not entirely a mainstream approach because the goals of reconstruction in the pediatric and adolescent patient are to preserve major rearfoot joint motion. In the cases of severe deformity where perfect postreconstruction alignment may not be achieved, it should be considered that improved alignment offers symptom resolution. Young patients may undergo osseous remodeling that may result in

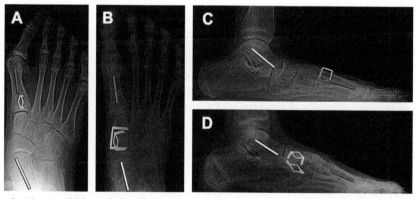

Fig. 9. 12-year-old boy, skeletally immature, with symptomatic flexible pes planus. (A, C) Preoperative weight-bearing images demonstrate multiplanar deformity. A retained staple is present from a failed previous epiphysiodesis for bunion correction. Note the significant medial column collapse with apex at the navicular cuneiform joint. (B, D) Healed postoperative weight-bearing images after navicular cuneiform fusion (with staples), first metatarsal closing base wedge, first metatarsal head osteotomy, medializing calcaneal osteotomy, and gastrocnemius recession. Restoration of proper talo-first metatarsal alignment (*yellow* and *blue lines*) is achieved. (*Courtesy of* Luke Cicchinelli, DPM, Mesa, AZ.)

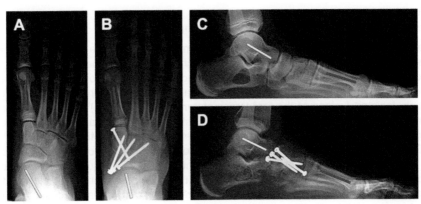

Fig. 10. 16-year-old boy, skeletally immature with near closed physis, with flexible pes planus who underwent reconstruction involving navicular cuneiform fusion. (*A, C*) Preoperative weight-bearing images demonstrate transverse plane deformity at the talonavicular joint (nearly 50% joint uncovering) and sagittal plane deformity (medial column collapse) with apex at the navicular cuneiform joint. An incidental benign calcaneal cyst is present. (*B, D*) Healed postoperative weight-bearing images after navicular cuneiform fusion is performed. Restoration of proper talo-first metatarsal alignment (*yellow* and *blue lines*) is achieved. Note that all 3 cuneiforms are incorporated into the fusion for the purpose of adducting and plantar flexing the midfoot to restore the arch. The return to talonavicular joint congruency is evident in the transverse plane, and illustrates the dramatic effect that a medial column fusion can have on the rearfoot complex. (*Courtesy of* Dan Choung, DPM, San Rafael, CA.)

improvement of the foot with time. Perhaps staged procedures can be considered with severe deformity. Rearfoot fusion is best indicated for the failed reconstruction.

SUMMARY

Pediatric and adolescent flexible flatfoot is a pathomechanically complex deformity. Conservative and surgical treatment is directed at realigning the foot and alleviating symptoms. When surgical intervention is considered, there are various methods and techniques that may be performed to realign the foot. A specific treatment algorithm does not exist, although planal dominance influences direct the surgeons when considering surgical intervention. Open physis often dictates the direction of the reconstruction. Attempts at essential joint preservation should be strongly considered in this young patient population.

REFERENCES

1. Cicchinelli LD, Pascual Huerta J, García Carmona FJ, et al. Analysis of gastrocnemius recession and medial column procedures as adjuncts in arthroereisis for the correction of pediatric pes planovalgus: a radiographic retrospective study. J Foot Ankle Surg 2008;47(5):385–91.
2. Kirby KA. The medial heel skive technique. Improving pronation control in foot orthoses. J Am Podiatr Med Assoc 1992;82(4):177–88.
3. Valmassy RL. Torsional and frontal plane conditions of the lower extremity. In: Thomson P, Volpe R, editors. Introduction to podopediatrics. 2nd edition. New York: Churchill Livingstone; 2001. p. 231–55.

4. Jay RM, Schoenhaus HD, Seymour C, et al. The dynamic stabilizing innersole system (DSIS): the management of hyperpronation in children. J Foot Ankle Surg 1995;34(2):124–31.
5. Logue JD. Advances in orthotics and bracing. Foot Ankle Clin 2007;12(2): 215–32.
6. Harris EJ, Vanore JV, Thomas JL. Diagnosis and treatment of pediatric flatfoot. J Foot Ankle Surg 2004;43(6):341–73.
7. el-Tayeby HM. The severe flexible flatfoot: a combined reconstructive procedure with rerouting of the tibialis anterior tendon. J Foot Ankle Surg 1999;38(1):41–9.
8. Lamm BM, Paley D, Herzenberg JE. Gastrocnemius soleus recession: a simpler, more limited approach. J Am Podiatr Med Assoc 2005;95(1):18–25.
9. Strayer LM Jr. Gastrocnemius recession; five-year report of cases. J Bone Joint Surg Am 1958;40(5):1019–30.
10. Strayer LM Jr. Recession of the gastrocnemius; an operation to relieve spastic contracture of the calf muscles. J Bone Joint Surg Am 1950;32(3):671–6.
11. Blitz NM, Eliot DJ. Anatomical aspects of the gastrocnemius aponeurosis and its insertion: a cadaveric study. J Foot Ankle Surg 2007;46(2):101–8.
12. Blitz NM, Eliot DJ. Anatomical aspects of the gastrocnemius aponeurosis and its muscular bound portion: a cadaveric study-part II. J Foot Ankle Surg 2008;47(6): 533–40.
13. Blitz NM, Rush SM. The gastrocnemius intramuscular aponeurotic recession: a simpli-fied method of gastrocnemius recession. J Foot Ankle Surg 2007;46(2):133–8.
14. Gourdine-Shaw MC, Lamm BM, Herzenberg JE, et al. Equinus deformity in the pediatric patient (etiology, evaluation, and management). Clin Podiatr Med Surg 2010;27(1):25–42.
15. DiDomenico LA, Adams HB, Garchar D. Endoscopic gastrocnemius recession for the treatment of gastrocnemius equinus. J Am Podiatr Med Assoc 2005; 95(4):410–3.
16. Vulpius O, Stoffel A. Orthopadische operationslehre. Stuttgart: Ferdinand Enke; 1913: 29–31.
17. Baker LD. Triceps surae syndrome in cerebral palsy; an operation to aid in its relief. Arch Surg 1954;68(2):216–21.
18. Chambers E. An operation for the correction of flexible flatfoot of adolescents. West J Surg Obstet Gynecol 1946;54:77–86.
19. Baker I, Hill L. Foot alignment in the cerebral palsy patient. J Bone Joint Surg Am 1964;46:1–15.
20. Selakovich W. Medial arch support by operation, sustentaculum tali procedure. Orthop Clin North Am 1973;4(1):117–44.
21. Giannini BS, Ceccarelli F, Benedetti MG, et al. Surgical treatment of flexible flatfoot in children, a four-year follow-up study. J Bone Joint Surg Am 2001; 83(Suppl 2 Pt 2):73–9.
22. Saxena A, Nguyen A. Preliminary radiographic findings and sizing implications on patients undergoing bioabsorbable subtalar arthroereisis. J Foot Ankle Surg 2007;46(3):175–80.
23. Needleman RL. A surgical approach for flexible flatfeet in adults including a sub-talar arthroereisis with the MBA sinus tarsi implant. Foot Ankle Int 2006;27(1): 9–18.
24. Kidner FC. The pre hallux (accessory scaphoid) in its relationship to flat foot. J Bone Joint Surg 1929;11:831.
25. Sullivan JA, Miller WA. The relationship of the accessory navicular to the develop-ment of the flat foot. Clin Orthop Relat Res 1979;144:233–7.

26. Chiu NT, Jou IM, Lee BF, et al. Symptomatic and asymptomatic accessory navicular bones: findings of Tc-99m MDP bone scintigraphy. Clin Radiol 2000;55(5):353–5.
27. Bennett GL, Weiner DS, Leighley B. Surgical treatment of symptomatic accessory tarsal navicular. J Pediatr Orthop 1990;10(4):445–9.
28. Kopp FJ, Marcus RE. Clinical outcome of surgical treatment of the symptomatic accessory navicular. Foot Ankle Int 2004;25(1):27–30.
29. Tan SM, Chin TW, Mitra AK, et al. Surgical treatment of symptomatic accessory navicular. Ann Acad Med Singap 1995;24(3):379–81.
30. Prichasuk S, Sinphurmsukskul O. Kidner procedure for symptomatic accessory navicular and its relation to pes planus. Foot Ankle Int 1995;16(8):500–3.
31. Knupp M, Hintermann B. The Cobb procedure for treatment of acquired flatfoot deformity associated with stage II insufficiency of the posterior tibial tendon. Foot Ankle Int 2007;28(4):416–21.
32. Baravarian B, Zgonis T, Lowery C. Use of the Cobb procedure in the treatment of posterior tibial tendon dysfunction. Clin Podiatr Med Surg 2002;19(3):371–89.
33. Benton-Weil W, Weil LS Jr. The Cobb procedure for stage II posterior tibial tendon dysfunction. Clin Podiatr Med Surg 1999;16(3):471–7.
34. Helal B. Cobb repair for tibialis posterior tendon rupture. J Foot Surg 1990;29(4):349–52.
35. Viegas GV. Reconstruction of the pediatric flexible planovalgus foot by using an Evans calcaneal osteotomy and augmentative medial split tibialis anterior tendon transfer. J Foot Ankle Surg 2003;42(4):199–207.
36. Young CS. Operative treatment of pes planus. Surg Gynecol Obstet 1939;68:1099–101.
37. Cohen-Sobel E, Giorgini R, Velez Z. Combined technique for surgical correction of pediatric severe flexible flatfoot. J Foot Ankle Surg 1995;34(2):183–94.
38. Dragonetti L, Ingraffia C, Stellari F. The Young tenosuspension in the treatment of abnormal pronation of the foot. J Foot Ankle Surg 1997;36(6):409–13.
39. Mosier-LaClair S, Pomeroy G, Manoli A 2nd. Operative treatment of the difficult stage 2 adult acquired flatfoot deformity. Foot Ankle Clin 2001;6(1):95–119.
40. Weinfeld SB. Medial slide calcaneal osteotomy. Technique, patient selection, and results. Foot Ankle Clin 2001;6(1):89–94.
41. Nyska M, Parks BG, Chu IT, et al. The contribution of the medial calcaneal osteotomy to the correction of flatfoot deformities. Foot Ankle Int 2001;22(4):278–82.
42. Catanzariti AR, Mendicino RW, King GL, et al. Double calcaneal osteotomy: realignment considerations in eight patients. J Am Podiatr Med Assoc 2005;95(1):53–9.
43. Weil LS Jr, Roukis TS. The calcaneal scarf osteotomy: operative technique. J Foot Ankle Surg 2001;40(3):178–82.
44. Dull JM, DiDomenico LA. Percutaneous displacement calcaneal osteotomy. J Foot Ankle Surg 2004;43(5):336–7.
45. Evans D. Calcaneo-valgus deformity. J Bone Joint Surg Br 1975;57:270–8.
46. Raines R, Brage M. Evans osteotomy in the adult foot: an anatomic study of structures at risk. Foot Ankle 1998;19:743–74.
47. Mosca V. Calcaneal lengthening for valgus deformity of the hindfoot. J Bone Joint Surg Am 1995;77:500–12.
48. Cooper PS, Nowak MD, Shaer J. Calcaneocuboid joint pressures with lateral column lengthening (Evans) procedure. Foot Ankle 1997;18:199–205.
49. DiNucci K, Christensen JC. Calcaneocuboid joint contact with Evans calcaneal osteotomy. In: Annual Meeting of the American College of Foot and Ankle Surgeons. San Francisco (CA), June 17–20, 1995.

50. Dinucci KR, Christensen JC, Dinucci KA. Biomechanical consequences of lateral column lengthening of the calcaneus: part I. Long plantar ligament strain. J Foot Ankle Surg 2004;43(1):10–5.
51. Tien TR, Parks BG, Guyton GP. Plantar pressures in the forefoot after lateral column lengthening: a cadaver study comparing the Evans osteotomy and calcaneocuboid fusion. Foot Ankle Int 2005;26(7):520–5.
52. Martin DE. Callus distraction: principles and indications. In: Banks AS, Downey MS, Martin DE, et al, editors. 3rd edition, McGlamry's comprehensive textbook of foot and ankle surgery, vol. 2. Philadelphia: Lippincott Williams and Wilkins; 2001. p. 2097–117.
53. Mosca VS. Calcaneal lengthening for valgus deformity of the hindfoot. Results in children who had severe, symptomatic flatfoot and skewfoot. J Bone Joint Surg Am 1995;77(4):500–12.
54. Davitt JS, MacWilliams BA, Armstrong PF. Plantar pressure and radiographic changes after distal calcaneal lengthening in children and adolescents. J Pediatr Orthop 2001;21(1):70–5.
55. Pomeroy GC, Manoli A 2nd. A new operative approach for flatfoot secondary to posterior tibial tendon insufficiency: a preliminary report. Foot Ankle Int 1997; 18(4):206–12.
56. Moseir-LaClair S, Pomeroy G, Manoli A 2nd. Intermediate follow-up on the double osteotomy and tendon transfer procedure for stage II posterior tibial tendon insufficiency. Foot Ankle Int 2001;22(4):283–91.
57. Cotton FJ. Foot statics and surgery. N Engl J Med 1936;214:353–62.
58. Helal B. Surgery for adolescent hallux valgus. Clin Orthop Relat Res 1981;157:50.
59. Kelikain H. Hallux valgus, allied deformities of the forefoot and metatarsalgia. Philadelphia: WB Saunders; 1965.
60. Young JD. A new operation for adolescent hallux valgus. Univ Pa Med Bull 1910; 23:459.
61. Fowler B, Brooks AL, Parrish TF. The cavovarus foot. J Bone Joint Surg Am 1959; 41:757.
62. Napiontek M, Kotwicki T, Tomaszewski M. Opening wedge osteotomy of the medial cuneiform before age 4 years in the treatment of forefoot adduction. J Pediatr Orthop 2003;23(1):65–9.
63. Lapidus PW. The operative correction of the metatarsus varus primus in hallux valgus. Surg Gynecol Obstet 1934;58:183–91.
64. Hoke M. An operation for the correction of extremely relaxed flatfeet. J Bone Joint Surg 1931;13:773–83.
65. Miller OL. A plastic flatfoot operation. J Bone Joint Surg 1927;9:84.
66. Dockery GL. Symptomatic juvenile flatfoot condition: surgical treatment. J Foot Ankle Surg 1995;34(2):135–45.

Rigid Pediatric Pes Planovalgus: Conservative and Surgical Treatment Options

Nitza Rodriguez, DPM[a],*, Danny J. Choung, DPM[b], Matthew B. Dobbs, MD[c]

KEYWORDS

- Rigid • Pediatric flatfoot • Pes planovalgus • Coalition
- Congenital vertical talus

Rigid pediatric pes planovalgus (RPPP), as the nomenclature states, refers to a condition of the foot in which the medial longitudinal arch height is abnormally decreased along with a significant loss of midfoot and hindfoot motion in the pediatric patient. Known causes for this condition are well documented and consist of congenital vertical talus, tarsal coalitions, and peroneal spastic flatfoot without coalition. Symptoms caused by RPPP typically involve pain or stiffness in the ankle, hindfoot, or midfoot. Timing of the symptoms may vary depending on the cause of the RPPP. Congenital vertical talus usually causes symptoms in early childhood due to the significant degree of deformity, which requires early intervention for correction. Otherwise, symptoms of RPPP can present during mid to late adolescence (especially in the case of tarsal coalitions) or adulthood or may never present at all.

CONGENITAL VERTICAL TALUS

Congenital vertical talus, also known as congenital convex pes valgus, is an uncommon rigid flatfoot deformity with severe hindfoot equinus and rocker-bottom structure. Its main features include a fixed dorsal dislocation of the navicular onto the talar neck while

[a] Northern California Foot and Ankle Center, 45 Castro Street, Suite 315, San Francisco, CA 94114, USA
[b] Department of Podiatric Surgery, Kaiser Permanente, 99 Monticello Road, San Rafael, CA 94903, USA
[c] Department of Orthopaedic Surgery, Washington University School of Medicine, One Children's Place, Suite 4S60, St Louis, MO 63110, USA
* Corresponding author.
E-mail address: nitzarodriguez@gmail.com (N. Rodriguez).

Clin Podiatr Med Surg 27 (2010) 79–92
doi:10.1016/j.cpm.2009.08.004
0891-8422/09/$ – see front matter
podiatric.theclinics.com

the talus is severely plantarflexed into a virtually vertical orientation.[1] Its incidence has been reported as 1 in 10,000.[2] Although half of the cases occur as an isolated deformity, the remaining cases involve neuromuscular and genetic disorders.[2–4]

At birth, the dorsal surface of the foot may contact the front of the tibia and can be confused with a calcaneovalgus foot deformity (**Fig. 1**). The plantar surface of the foot is convex, with a prominent talar head at the medial plantar aspect of the longitudinal arch. The hindfoot is in severe equinovalgus due to the contractures of the gastrocnemius-soleus complex, tibialis anterior, extensor hallucis longus, and the peroneal tendons, leaving the forefoot abducted, dorsiflexed, and everted.

The natural history of an untreated vertical talus is one of significant disability. Patients have poor push-off and are forced to weight bear on the talar head. This leads to painful callosities and abnormal shoe wear. Gait can be awkward long-term with many patients having difficulty with balance.[5]

The exact cause of vertical talus in many cases is not known but a genetic basis seems likely. There is a positive family history in 12% to 20% of patients with idiopathic vertical talus. In those with a family history, the deformity is inherited in an autosomal dominant fashion with incomplete penetrance. A mutation in the HOXD10 gene is responsible for vertical talus in some familial cases but not all.[6,7] HOX genes are a large group of highly conserved transcription factors that control development along the body axis.

Another gene identified for vertical talus is the cartilage-derived morphogenetic protein-1 gene (CDMP-1).[8] Mutations in CDMP-1 have also been described in Grebe and Hunter-Thompson forms of acromelic skeletal dysplasia and Du Pan syndrome; these syndromes present with severe limb abnormalities.

RADIOGRAPHIC EVALUATION

Stress plantarflexion and stress dorsiflexion lateral views confirm the diagnosis. The former demonstrates the irreducibility of the talonavicular joint and hindfoot equinus, as the talar axis passes far plantar to the first metatarsal axis. The latter reveals the rigidly fixed hindfoot equinus. The line bisecting the talus is almost vertical, nearly paralleling the tibia, whereas the calcaneus is in equinus and the forefoot is dorsiflexed (**Fig. 2**).

CONSERVATIVE AND SURGICAL TREATMENT
Surgical History of Congenital Vertical Talus

The essential goal of treatment is to restore the anatomic relationship of the navicular, talus, and calcaneus as soon as possible. Early treatments of idiopathic congenital

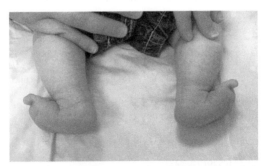

Fig. 1. Bilateral congenital vertical talus. Note the dorsal surface of the foot is in contact with the anterior tibia and the rocker-bottom shape of the feet.

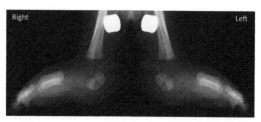

Fig. 2. Bilateral congenital vertical talus. Preoperative Dobbs and colleagues reduction films. Note the talar axis passes plantar to the first metatarsal axis and the bisection of the talus is almost vertical, nearly paralleling the tibia, while the calcaneus is in equinus and the forefoot is dorsiflexed.

vertical talus were manipulation and casting. Many reported failed corrections, usually resulting in reconstructive surgery.[3,9–17] Radical early surgical procedures consisted of excision of the talus or navicular.[1,13] The trend then moved toward staged, two-incision reconstructive surgery.[12,18,19] The high incidence of complications noted with these techniques gave rise to several single-stage surgical approaches.[20,21] In recent literature, a single-stage dorsal approach was described by Seimon, who advocated tenotomizing the extensor hallucis longus and peroneus tertius, open reduction of the talonavicular joint with Kirschner (K)–wire fixation, and percutaneous Achilles tendon lengthening.[22] Other investigators have also reported good results and fewer complications with this technique.[16,23]

In 2006, Dobbs and colleagues came full circle when they published their early results of a new method of treatment consisting of serial manipulations and casting based on the principles of the Ponseti treatment of clubfoot.[24] All components of the deformity are addressed simultaneously except the equinus, which is corrected last.

Dobbs and Colleagues' Conservative Method of Treatment of Congenital Vertical Talus

Treatment is initiated if possible in the first few weeks of life. The series of weekly long leg cast applications begin with gentle manipulations and stretching. The foot is adducted and plantarflexed while counter pressure is applied medially to the talar head. All components of the vertical talus are corrected simultaneously with manipulation with the exception of the hindfoot equinus, which is corrected last. After a few minutes of gentle manipulations, a long leg cast is applied. The cast is applied in two sections, the first of which is applied as a short leg plaster cast while the foot is plantarflexed and inverted and the second an extension into a long leg cast with the knee in 90° of flexion. It is important to apply the cast in two sections to focus on molding the foot in the short leg portion of the cast. The final cast, which is usually the fifth casting session, is applied with the foot in maximum plantarflexion and inversion, resembling a clubfoot, to insure adequate stretching of all the dorsolateral soft tissues. A lateral radiograph is taken of this final cast to assess proper reduction of the talonavicular joint. (In maximum plantarflexion, the talar axis–first metatarsal base angle should be <30°.)

Once the talonavicular joint is reduced, patients are scheduled for surgery for pin fixation of the talonavicular joint and a percutaneous Achilles tendon tenotomy. In the operating room, the foot is held in plantarflexion and a radiograph is used to confirm reduction. A small skin incision is then made on the medial aspect of the foot over the talonavicular joint. If the joint is already reduced, the skin incision allows direct visualization of the talus and navicular for correct K-wire placement. This is important as the bones are difficult to palpate in a young child and can lead to erroneous wire placement. A K-wire is placed retrograde from the navicular into the talus. The wire is cut and left buried underneath the skin to prevent the wire from backing out.

If the talonavicular joint is not reduced all the way with casting, then a small dorsal capsulotomy is performed to complete the reduction. The capsulotomy is performed through the same medial skin incision described previously. Rarely the peroneus brevis tendon or the tibialis anterior tendon is fractionally lengthened at the musculotendinous junction if determined to be impeding reduction. For patients older than 2 years at the time of treatment, the proximal half of the tibialis anterior tendon is transferred to the dorsal aspect of the neck of the talus to act as a sling and a dynamic corrective force. Once talonavicular stabilization is achieved, percutaneous tenotomy of the Achilles tendon is done for correction of the equinus.[25] A long leg cast is then worn for 2 weeks with the foot in neutral position and ankle in 5° of dorsiflexion. The cast is changed in the operating room 2 weeks later to assess motion and pin placement with a radiograph. Patients are also measured for a nighttime brace that consists of an articulating bar with custom-molded orthoses that keep the feet in neutral position.[26] The bar allows for independent leg movement while the custom orthoses hold the feet in the desired position. For syndromic and neuromuscular vertical talus patients, solid ankle foot orthosis are used for daytime and ambulation in addition to the nighttime brace wear. After brace measurement, a new long leg cast is applied with 10° to 15° of ankle dorsiflexion for 4 weeks, after which the K-wire is removed and the brace is fit. The nighttime bracing is used for 2 years.

A small short-term study done by Bhaskar also reported promising results based on the same principles described by Dobbs and colleagues.[27] Long-term studies are necessary to assess maintenance of reduction (**Fig. 3**). The authors anticipate that, like the Ponseti method for clubfoot treatment, this less invasive method for vertical talus will lead to more functional and mobile feet in the long-term while avoiding the complication of extensive soft-tissue release surgeries.[28] The upper age limit for this technique is yet to be defined but it is currently being used successfully on older children.

TARSAL COALITIONS

Tarsal coalition is defined as an abnormal union between two or more bones in the hindfoot or midfoot. This union may be complete or incomplete giving rise to three types of coalitions: fibrous (syndesmosis), cartilaginous (synchondrosis), or osseous (synostosis). Although most rigid flatfeet are attributed to tarsal coalitions, some

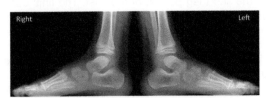

Fig. 3. Bilateral congenital vertical talus 5 years status post Dobbs and colleagues reduction (serial casting, talonavicular joint K-wire stabilization, and percutaneous tenotomy of the Achilles tendon) films. Note the drastic improvement in the alignment of the talar axis, which now is in line with the first metatarsal axis.

coalitions may occur in the presence of a normally aligned or a cavus-type foot. Reported incidence of tarsal coalitions ranges from 0.04% to 1.4%.[29-31]

The condition is believed congenital and caused by a genetic mutation to an autosomal dominant gene resulting in failure of differentiation and segmentation of primitive mesenchyme.[32-43] Acquired tarsal coalitions also have been described, arising from trauma, infection, surgery, neoplasms, ossicle incorporation, or articular disorders.[44] These are rarely seen in pediatric patients.[45]

Calcaneonavicular and talocalcaneal middle facet coalitions account for 90% of all coalitions, both occurring with equal frequency and approximately 50% of cases occurring bilaterally.[46] Other tarsal coalitions are described, consisting of calcaneocuboid, talonavicular, intercuneiform, naviculocuneiform, cubonavicular, and cubocuneiform coalitions.

Symptoms related to tarsal coalition typically present during mid to late adolescence, when the coalition ossifies,[47] and usually involve hindfoot pain about the sustentaculum tali or sinus tarsi or referred pain to the leg.[48] The symptoms are believed related to significant limitation of normal hindfoot range of motion, associated flatfoot deformity, or secondary arthritic changes. Symptoms can often develop insidiously after minor trauma or excessive weight-bearing activity. Tarsal coalitions also are reported as associated with more frequent ankle sprains in an active teenager.[47,49]

Physical examination reveals limited hindfoot range of motion, especially in the frontal plane. Varying degrees of pes planus deformity are frequently associated with calcaneonavicular or talocalcaneal coalitions. Gastrocnemius or gastrosoleal equinus of the ankle also accompany the rigid pes planus deformity in the majority of cases. The historical classic finding of peroneal spasticity is not as common as once thought and should not be considered pathognomonic for a tarsal coalition.[50] When such a finding is present, however, it is thought to be a guarding reflex to the limited subtalar joint range of motion.

When assessing the subtalar joint range of motion, it is important to lock up the ankle mortise by dorsiflexing the tibiotalar joint to avoid any false sense of adequate frontal plane subtalar joint motion that may occur through the ankle joint. The ankle joint may have increased frontal plane range of motion due to compensatory adaptation or lateral ligamentous laxity that is often associated with rigid pes planus deformities.

The location of pain varies depending on the type of coalition. In patients with a calcaneonavicular bar, the pain is usually located at the sinus tarsi due to the proximity of the calcaneonavicular junction. In one with a middle facet talocalcaneal coalition, the pain is consistently located at the sinus tarsi and over the sustentaculum tali, which is often overly prominent. Both, however, can have pain in similar locations or diffuse pain about the hindfoot.

RADIOGRAPHIC EVALUATION

Radiographic evaluation begins with proper plain film radiographs, and the coalition itself or secondary radiographic features common to all three types of rearfoot coalitions can often be identified: talonavicular (**Fig. 4**), calcaneonavicular (**Fig. 5**), and talocalcaneal (**Fig. 6**). The medial-oblique (or 45° oblique) view best demonstrates a calcaneonavicular coalition (see **Fig. 5**A), whereas the lateral and Harris-Beath views best reveal a middle facet coalition (see **Fig. 6**B). Secondary signs are well described. Talar beaking, seen on the lateral view, suggests increased capsuloligamentous traction on the superior aspect of the talar head resulting from compensatory mechanical demands at the talonavicular joint. The halo or C sign, a circular density seen on the

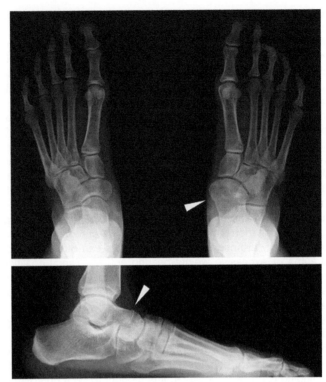

Fig. 4. Incomplete congenital talonavicular joint coalition (*arrowhead*) in a 17-year-old girl's right foot.

lateral view about the sustentaculum tali, suggests middle facet talocalcaneal coalition. The anteater nose sign (see **Fig. 5**B) is associated with calcaneonavicular coalitions and is seen as an elongation of the anterior-superior process of the calcaneus.[51] Other secondary radiographic findings include broadening or rounding of the

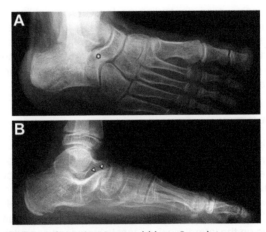

Fig. 5. Calcaneonavicular coalition in 10-year-old boy. Complete osseous coalition between calcaneus and navicular (*asterisk*) best visualized on medial oblique view (*A*) and anteater sign seen on lateral view (*B*).

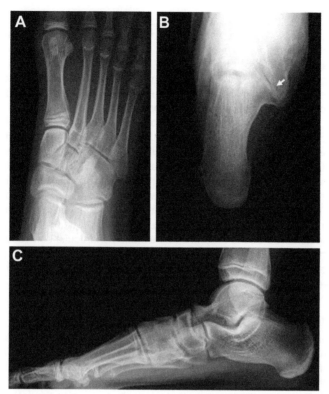

Fig. 6. Symptomatic rigid pes planus in a 14-year-old boy secondary to middle facet tarsal coalition. (*A, C*) A pes planus deformity is evident with significant lateral peritalar subluxation, nonarthritic dorsal talonavicular joint beaking, and broadening of the lateral talar process. (*B*) Harris-Beath radiographs clearly identify the characteristic obliquity of the middle facet in a medial-plantar orientation (*arrow*). This is particular coalition is a fibrous coalition.

lateral talar process, narrowing of the posterior subtalar joint, and ball-and-socket appearance of the tibiotalar joint on an anterior-posterior plain ankle radiograph.

CT, the gold standard in imaging tarsal coalitions, demonstrates type of coalition (osseous vs nonosseous), extent of coalition (especially in talocalcaneal coalitions), and secondary degenerative joint changes. Its application is best suited for middle facet talocalcaneal coalitions, which have varied presentations (see **Fig. 6**). In the nonosseous type, there usually is significant narrowing and irregularity of the joint and sustentacular and corresponding talar hypertrophy. The joint is often oblique toward a medial plantar direction. These CT scan findings and considerations are instrumental in surgical planning.

CONSERVATIVE AND SURGICAL TREATMENTS

The goal of conservative treatment is to restrict subtalar and midtarsal joint range of motion in an effort to reduce pain and muscle spasms. These measures consist of custom orthosis, shoe modifications, and immobilization with cast, splints, or crutches. If conservative measures fail, then surgical treatment is indicated. The surgical approach is dependent on the type of coalition and age of the child.

Calcaneonavicular Coalitions

Traditionally, pediatric patients with symptomatic calcaneonavicular coalitions have been surgically treated with resection soon after the symptoms arise, especially if no degenerative changes or other coalitions are present. During the surgical procedure, attention should be taken to avoid injuring the intermediate or lateral dorsal cutaneous nerves. The extensor digitorum brevis muscle belly is identified and its origin is reflected exposing the coalition, which is then resected in a rectangular fashion. It is important to maximize the resection while avoiding harm to the talonavicular or calcaneocuboid joints, which can be achieved with the use of intraoperative fluoroscopy. The resection can be performed with an oscillating saw or an osteotome. The depth of the resection is usually more extensive than anticipated. If using a saw, an osteotome can be used to finish the resection to help prevent needless soft tissue injury. At this point, the gap may be interposed with soft tissue (eg, extensor digitorum muscle belly) or bone wax applied to the resected bone surfaces to minimize osseous regeneration. The range of motion that is acquired varies, but full range of motion may not always be achieved due to the limits of the static periarticular soft tissues or adaptations within the joint. When calcaneonavicular coalitions are present with a significant pes planus deformity, mere resection might not be adequate and the flat foot deformity may need to be addressed.

Talocalcaneal Coalitions

The treatment of middle facet talocalcaneal coalitions continues to be a topic of debate. In the past, surgical treatment consisted of resection of the coalition with or without hindfoot arthrodeses. Isolated resection of the coalition is generally limited to younger patients without significant flatfoot deformity and secondary degenerative changes.[52–55] Recent studies propose that surgically addressing the flatfoot deformity in cases without secondary arthrosis would result in better outcomes.[54,56–58] Kernbach and colleagues advocate single-stage middle facet coalition resection combined with flatfoot reconstruction based on their surgical experiences with six patients.[56]

Other studies have focused on the extent of the coalition, suggesting better outcomes when the coalition involves one third or less of the total surface area of the middle facet of the subtalar joint on CT. Extent of coalition has not been correlated in outcome measures, however.[58,59] Some investigators have proposed isolated subtalar joint arthrodesis, reasoning that motion saved in the midtarsal joints would better preserve load transfer, thereby slowing the progression of degenerative changes in adjacent joints.[60] Nonetheless, in cases of overt arthrosis of the subtalar and the talonavicular joints, triple arthrodesis seems to remain the choice procedure.

Surgical treatment of a rigid flatfoot with talocalcaneal coalition requires careful review of symptoms. A thorough physical examination determines if the causes of the symptoms are related solely to the coalition, secondary arthritic changes, pes planus deformity, or any combinations thereof.[56] Surgical decisions should be based on areas of tenderness, degree of flatfoot deformity and ankle equinus, amount of midtarsal flexibility, and careful analysis of radiographic studies.

In the presence of severe pes planus, mere resection may lead to increase pronatory forces through the subtalar joint potentially increasing the deformity and symptoms. Along with any structurally corrective procedures, addressing the ankle equinus (whether by gastrocnemius recession or tendo-Achilles lengthening) should be fundamental, because it is a major pronatory deforming force to the foot.[61]

In the absence of symptoms originating from arthritic changes, the goal is to reduce the deformity while preserving the essential hindfoot joints.[61] This maintains the dampening effects of the talonavicular and subtalar joints throughout the gait cycle, thereby minimizing mechanical overload of neighboring joints, which leads to secondary arthritis. Bone-block distraction osteotomy of the anterior calcaneus (ie, the Evans osteotomy),[62] medially displacing osteotomy of the posterior calcaneus (ie, the Koutsogiannis osteotmoy),[63] naviculocuneiform joint arthrodesis, subtalar ar- throereisis, and first metatarsocuneiform joint arthrodesis (if the proximal physis has closed) all are surgical procedures that may be used to correct the pes planus defor- mity while sparing the essential hindfoot joints. Usually a combination of these proce- dures may be required with optional supplemental soft tissue procedures (eg, posterior tibial tendon augmentation or Young's tenosuspension). Recently, a treat- ment algorithm for flatfoot reconstruction combined with coalition resection has been proposed.[56]

In the rigid flatfoot, the intended effects of these procedures may often be better determined intraoperatively after the coalition has been resected and the resulting hindfoot range of motion can be assessed. Mere resection of the coalition in the absence of arthritis does not automatically convert the rigid flatfoot into a flexible one. Depending on the age of the patient, extent of the coalition, and adaptations (eg, molding of the talar head), the obtained subtalar joint range of motion may be variably less than anticipated, rendering the foot less amenable to such aforemen- tioned procedures. Several published reports suggest the benefit, however, of surgi- cally addressing the flatfoot deformity without hindfoot arthrodeses in rigid flatfoot secondary to talocalcaneal coalitions.[48,56,64–66] Recently, in the absence of concom- itant rearfoot arthrosis, Kernbach and colleagues reported on single-stage flatfoot reconstruction involving a varying combination (naviculocuneiform joint arthrodesis, Evans calcaneal osteotomy, medializing calcaneal osteotomy, Achilles lengthening/ gastrocnemius recession, and posterior tibial tendon augmentation) with middle facet talocalcaneal coalition resection, demonstrating statistically improved postop- erative radiographic angular corrections.[56] This method was proposed for varying degrees of rigid pes planus, in which the deformity likely contributes to the symp- toms, with the implication that this combined approach may obviate or delay future hindfoot arthrosis. Long-term studies are required to help substantiate their tentative conclusions.

In the arthritic subtalar joint, hindfoot fusion is unquestionably required. An isolated subtalar joint arthrodesis may not suffice, however, in correcting the entire flatfoot deformity, especially in the presence of significant midtarsal abduction or sagittal instability of the medial column. Although triple arthrodesis has historically been advocated in these circumstances, concern for future ankle or midfoot arthrosis may argue toward midfoot fusion (naviculocuneiform or first metatarsocu- neiform joint arthrodesis), depending on the apex of the medial column deformity or instability. It is the authors' opinion that a naviculocuneiform joint arthrodesis can closely restore normal talo–first metatarsal angle, as measured in the dorsal-to- plantar and lateral radiographs, in cases where the dorsolateral peritalar subluxation does not uncover more than 40% to 50% of the medial talar head (Fig. 7). Adequate débridement of the joint, including all the cuneiforms, increases its flexibility to allow for significant adduction, plantarflexion or plantar translation, and valgus rotation of the medial column, which can largely contribute to restoring the arch. In addition, arthrodesis of this joint is preferable because in most cases the first metatarsal physis still is open, obviating the option for a first metatarsocuneiform joint arthrod- esis. In deformities where the medial talar head is uncovered more than 40% or overt arthrosis exists in the midtarsal joints, triple arthrodesis may be better indicated.

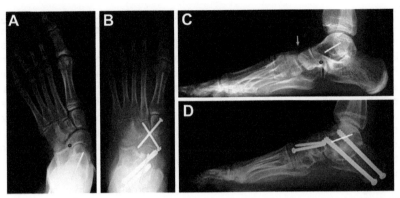

Fig. 7. Single-stage flatfoot reconstruction combined with talocalcaneal and calcaneonavicular coalition resection in 15-year-old girl. (*A, C*) Preoperative weight-bearing radiographs demonstrate calcaneonavicular coalition (*red asterisk*) and talocalcaneal coalition with significant pes planus with naviculocuneiform fault (*green arrow*). (*B, D*) Postoperative weight-bearing radiographs after resection of both coalitions, gastrocnemius recession, and subtalar and navicular joint arthrodesis. Improved talo–first metatarsal angle (*yellow and blue lines*) is evident. Foot is realigned without resorting to triple arthrodesis.

OTHER ETIOLOGIES OF RIGID FLATFOOT

Other potential causes of RPPP include iatrogenic deformities and peroneal spastic flatfoot without coalition. Iatrogenic rigid flatfoot deformities, although uncommon, may result from overcorrected clubfoot, undercorrected vertical talus, failed flatfoot surgery, and end-stage trauma.[67] Peroneal spastic flatfoot without coalition may occur for a variety of reasons, including pain, trauma, infection, or arthritis of the hindfoot joints.[68–70] Common peroneal nerve block has been advocated for peroneal spastic flatfoot in the presence or absence of tarsal coalition to allow better assessment of motion.[69] Although a comprehensive discussion of these origins is beyond the focus of this article, these deformities are complex and require extensive diagnostic work-up and possible revisional surgery.

SUMMARY

RPPP is a condition of the foot causing significant disability due to loss of midfoot and hindfoot motion. Appropriate diagnosis and treatment is imperative to improve the quality of life in these patients.

Surgical treatment of RPPP is a variegated topic due to different causes and multiple surgical approaches. The foot is a complex biomechanical structure that not only supports the entire body but also functions intricately to dampen the forces transmitted through locomotion. Form and function mutually play an important role in this respect. In the rigid pes planovalgus, deformity precedes dysfunction and, undoubtedly, the form needs to be restored for suitable function. Several conservative and surgical procedures and approaches are discussed.

There seems to be a proclivity toward maximizing natural foot biomechanics that translates to sparing the essential hindfoot joints. This is demonstrated in the treatment of congenital vertical talus, where a paradigm shift has occurred from radical surgical treatment to serial casting in combination with minimally invasive procedures. This drastic correction of the deformity without arthrodesis or excision of bone allows for the best physiologic biomechanical function.

In tarsal coalitions associated with rigid pes planus, emphasis is also placed on preserving hindfoot range of motion once the coalition is resected. Surgical procedures for flexible pes planus have been applied to tarsal coalitions with rigid pes planus without concomitant arthritis. Additional considerations regarding preoperative and intraoperative planning are necessary when dealing with RPPP, however. This is because a resected coalition frequently does not result in a pes planus with characteristics equivalent to a flexible type. Therefore, surgeons should be prepared intraoperatively to modify the combination of reconstructive procedures or perhaps consider selective hindfoot arthrodeses along with other hindfoot or midfoot procedures.

These considerations demonstrate a fine line between restoring foot structure and maximizing foot function that needs careful attention and skillful management to arrive at the best outcome in the treatment of RPPP. Keeping the essential hindfoot joints intact is preferable but not at the cost of inadequately reducing the deformity. This discussion, especially regarding tarsal coalitions, requires further substantiation with long-term studies.

ACKNOWLEDGMENTS

We would like to thank our families and colleagues who have supported us in this process, in particular Dr Neal Blitz. This article is dedicated to our patients who inspire us to seek ways of improving their quality of life.

REFERENCES

1. Lamy L, Weissman L. Congenital convex pes valgus. J Bone Joint Surg Am 1939; 21:79–90.
2. Jacobsen ST, Crawford AH. Congenital vertical talus. J Pediatr Orthop 1983;3: 306–10.
3. Dodge LD, Ashley RK, Gilbert RJ. Treatment of the congenital vertical talus: a retrospective review of 36 feet with long-term follow-up. Foot Ankle 1987;7: 326–32.
4. Hamanishi C. Congenital vertical talus: classification with 69 cases and new measurement system. J Pediatr Orthop 1984;4:318–26.
5. Alaee F, Boehm S, Dobbs MB. A new approach to the treatment of congenital vertical talus. J Child Orthop 2007;1:165–74.
6. Dobbs MB, Gurnett CA, Pierce B, et al. HOXD10 M319K Mutation in a family with isolated congenital vertical talus. J Orthop Res 2006;24(3):448–53.
7. Gurnett CA, Keppel C, Bick J, et al. Absence of HOXD10 Mutations in idiopathic clubfoot and sporadic vertical talus. Clin Orthop Relat Res 2007;462:27–31.
8. Dobbs MB, Gurnett C, Robarge J, et al. Variable hand and foot abnormalities in family with congenital vertical talus and CDMP-1 gene mutation. J Orthop Res 2005;23(6):1490–4.
9. Drennan JC, Sharrard WJ. The pathological anatomy of convex pes valgus. J Bone Joint Surg Br 1971;53:455–61.
10. Colton CL. The surgical management of congenital vertical talus. J Bone Joint Surg Br 1973;55:566–74.
11. Ellis JN, Scheer GE. Congenital convex pes valgus. Clin Orthop Relat Res 1974; 99:168–74.
12. Coleman SS, Stelling FH 3rd, Jarrett J. Pathomechanics and treatment of congenital vertical talus. Clin Orthop 1970;70:62–72.
13. Erye-Brook AL. Congenital vertical talus. J Bone Joint Surg Br 1967;49:618–27.

14. Eraltug U. Corrective plaster application in the treatment of vertical talus. An analysis of eleven cases. Int Surg 1997;18:535–43.
15. Griffin DW, Daly N, Karlin JM. Clinical presentation of congenital convex pes valgus. J Foot Ankle Surg 1995;34:146–52.
16. Stricker SJ, Rosen E. Early one-stage reconstruction of congenital vertical talus. Foot Ankle Int 1997;18:535–43.
17. Becker-Anderson H, Reimann I. Congenital vertical talus. Reevaluation of early manipulation treatment. Acta Orthop Scand 1974;45:130–44.
18. Osmond-Clarke H. Congenital vertical talus. J Bone Joint Surg Br 1956;38(1): 33–41.
19. Herndon CH, Heyman CH. Problems in the recognition and treatment of congenital pes valgus. J Bone Joint Surg Am 1963;45:413–29.
20. Ogata K, Schoenecker PL, Sheridan J. Congenital vertical talus and its familial occurrence: an analysis of 36 patients. Clin Orthop 1979;139:128–32.
21. Kodros SA, Dias LS. Single-stage surgical correction of congenital vertical talus. J Pediatr Orthop 1999;19:42–8.
22. Seimon LP. Surgical correction of congenital vertical talus under the age of 2 years. J Pediatr Orthop 1987;7:405–11.
23. Mazzocca AD, Thomson JD, Deluca PA, et al. Comparison of the posterior approach versus the dorsal approach in the treatment of congenital vertical talus. J Pediatr Orthop 2001;21:212–7.
24. Ponseti IV. Treatment of congenital club foot. J Bone Joint Surg 1992;74(3): 448–54.
25. Dobbs MB, Gordon JE, Walton T, et al. Bleeding complications following percutaneous tendo-Achilles tenotomy in the treatment of clubfoot deformity. J Pediatr Orthop 2004;24:353–7.
26. Matthew B. Dobbs/The Miller Group. Dobbs Dynamic Clubfoot Brace. Available at: dobbsbrace.com. Accessed January 5, 2009.
27. Bhaskar A. Congenital vertical talus: treatment by reverse ponseti technique. Indian J Orthop 2008;42:347–50.
28. Dobbs MB, Nunley R, Schoenecker PL. Long-term follow-up of patients with clubfeet treated with extensive soft-tissue release. J Bone Joint Surg 2006;88(5): 986–96.
29. Rankin EA, Baker GI. Rigid flatfoot in the young adult. Clin Orthop 1974;104: 244–8.
30. Shands AR Jr, Wentz IJ. Congenital anomalies, accessory bones, and osteochondritis in the feet of 850 children. Surg Clin North Am 1953;33:1643–66.
31. Vaughan WH, Segal G. Tarsal coalition, with special reference to roentgenographic interpretation. Radiology 1953;60:855–63.
32. Leonard MA. The inheritance of tarsal coalition and its relationship to spastic flat foot. J Bone Joint Surg 1974;56:520–6.
33. Barsani FA, Samilson RL. Massive familial tarsal synostosis. J Bone Joint Surg 1957;39:1187–90.
34. Boyd HB. Congenital talonavicular synostosis. J Bone Joint Surg 1944;26: 682–6.
35. Glessner JR Jr, Davis GL. Bilateral calcaneonavicular coalition occurring in twin boys: a case study. Clin Orthop 1966;47:173–6.
36. Hodgson FG. Talonavicular synostosis. Southampt Med J 1946;39:940–1.
37. Downey MS. Tarsal coalition. In: McGlamry ED, Banks AS, Downey MS, editors. Comprehensive textbook of foot surgery. 3rd edition. Philadelphia: Williams & Watkins; 2001. p. 993–1027.

38. Pensieri SL, Jay RM, Schoenhaus HD, et al. Bilateral congenital calcaneocuboid synostosis and subtalar joint coalition. J Am Podiatr Med Assoc 1985; 75:406–10.
39. Plotkin S. Case presentation of calcaneonavicular coalition in monozygotic twins. J Am Podiatr Med Assoc 1996;86:433–8.
40. Rothberg AS, Feldman JW, Schuster OF. Congenital fusion of astragalus and scaphoid: bilateral; inherited. N Y State J Med 1935;35:29–31.
41. Webster FS, Roberts WM. Tarsal anomalies and peroneal spastic flatfoot. JAMA 1951;146:1099–104.
42. Wray JB, Herndon CN. Hereditary transmission of congenital coalition of the calcaneus to the navicular. J Bone Joint Surg 1963;45:365–72.
43. Kumai T, Takakura Y, Akiyama K, et al. Histopathological study of nonosseous tarsal coalition. Foot Ankle Int 1998;19:525–31.
44. Page JC. Peroneal spastic flatfoot and tarsal coalition. J Am Podiatr Med Assoc 1987;77:29–34.
45. Downey MS. Resection of middle facet talocalcaneal coalitions. In: Miller SJ, Mahan KT, Yu GV, et al, editors. Reconstructive surgery of the foot and leg: update '98. Tucker (GA): Podiatry Institute; 1998. p. 1–5.
46. Stormont DM, Peterson HA. The relative incidence of tarsal coalition. Clin Orthop 1983;181:28–36.
47. Cowell HR, Elener V. Rigid painful flatfoot secondary to tarsal coalition. Clin Orthop 1983;177:54–60.
48. Giannini S, Ceccarelli F, Vannini F, et al. Operative treatment of flatfoot with talocalcaneal coalition. Clin Orthop Relat Res 2003;411:178–87.
49. Morgan RC Jr, Crawford AH. Surgical management of tarsal coalition in adolescent athletes. Foot Ankle 1986;7:183–93.
50. Bohne WH. Tarsal coalition. Curr Opin Pediatr 2001;13(1):29–35.
51. Kulik SA, Clanton TO. Tarsal coalition. Foot Ankle Int 1996;17(5):286–96.
52. Herzenberg JE, Goldner JL, Martinez S, et al. Computerized tomography of talocalcaneal tarsal coalition: a clinical and anatomic study. Foot Ankle 1986;66: 273–88.
53. Raikin S, Cooperman DR, Thompson GH. Interposition of the Split flexor hallucis longus tendon after resection of a coalition of the middle facet of the talocalcaneal joint. J Bone Joint Surg 1999;811:11–9.
54. Rouvreau P, Pouliquen JC, Langlais J, et al. Synostosis and tarsal coalitions in children. A study of 68 cases in 47 patients. Rev Chir Orthop Reparatrice Appar Mot 1994;803:252–60.
55. Salter RB. Congenital abnormalities. In: Textbook of disorders and injuries of the musculoskeletal system. 3rd edition. Baltimore: Lippincott, Williams and Wilkins; 1999. p. 141–2.
56. Kernbach KJ, Blitz NM, Rush SM. Bilateral single stage middle facet coalition resection combined with flatfoot reconstruction. A report of 3 cases. Investigations involving middle facet coalitions—part I. J Foot Ankle Surg 2008;47:180–90.
57. Luhmann SJ, Schoenecker PL. Symptomatic talocalcaneal coalition resection: indications and results. J Pediatr Orthop 1998;186:748–54.
58. Wilde PH, Torode IP, Dickens DR, et al. Resection for symptomatic talocalcaneal coalition. J Bone Joint Surg Br 1994;76:797–801.
59. Comfort TK, Johnson LO. Resection for symptomatic talocalcaneal coalition. J Pediatr Orthop 1998;18(3):283–8.
60. Mann RA, Baumgarten M. Subtalar fusion for isolated subtalar disorders. Preliminary report. Clin Orthop 1988;226:260–5.

61. Hansen ST. Progressive symptomatic flatfoot. In: Functional reconstruction of the foot and ankle. Philadelphia: Lippincott, Williams and Wilkins; 2000. p. 24–5.

62. Evans D. Calcaneovalgus deformity. J Bone Joint Surg Br 1975;57:270–8.

63. Koutsogiannis E. Treatment of mobile flat foot by displacement osteotomy of the calcaneus. J Bone Joint Surg Br 1971;53(1):96–100.

64. Yen RG, Giacopelli JA, Granoff DP, et al. New nonfusion procedure for talocalcaneal coalitions with a fixed heel valgus. J Am Podiatr Med Assoc 1993;83:191–7.

65. Lepow GM, Richman HM. Talocalcaneal coalition: a unique treatment approach in case report. Podiatry Tracts 1988;1:38–43.

66. Collins B. Tarsal coalitions. A new surgical procedure. Clin Podiatr Med Surg 1987;41:75–98.

67. Harris E, Vanore J, Thomas J, et al. Diagnosis and treatment of pediatric flatfoot: clinical practice guideline. J Foot Ankle Surg 2004;43(6):341–73.

68. Blair J, Perdios A, Reilly C. Peroneal spastic flatfoot caused by osteochondral lesion: a case report. Foot Ankle Int 2007;28(6):724–6.

69. Lowy LJ. Pediatric peroneal spastic flatfoot in the absence of coalition: a suggested protocol. J Am Podiatr Med Assoc 1998;88:181–91.

70. Mosier KM, Asher M. Tarsal coalitions and peroneal spastic flatfoot: a review. J Bone Joint Surg Am 1984;66:976–84.

Pediatric Metatarsus Adductus and Skewfoot Deformity

Byron Hutchinson, DPM, FACFAS[a,b,c,*]

KEYWORDS

- Skewfoot • Flatfoot • Pediatric deformities
- Surgical management

Metatarsus adductus as an isolated deformity is a well-known clinical entity and, with early recognition, clinical outcomes have been desirable.[1–3] The vast majority of these deformities respond to nonoperative therapy.[1,4] A long-standing untreated or under-treated metatarsus adductus can lead to the formation of a skewfoot deformity that can have very significant symptoms and less successful treatment by nonoperative means.[5] The pathogenesis of skewfoot is unknown and there is no reported post-mortem analysis of skewfoot. In 1986, a prospective study by Berg[6] of 124 feet showed that those patients with a skewfoot deformity required cast immobilization twice as long as those with simple metatarsus adductus.

The term skewfoot has been misrepresented in the literature resulting in some confusion about the deformity itself. McCormick and Blount[7] coined the term skewfoot in 1949 as another way of representing metatarsus adductus. Most authors today define skewfoot simply as forefoot adduction and heel valgus. Synonyms include S-shaped foot, serpentine foot, and Z-foot deformities.[8] There is a paucity of literature dealing with diagnosis and management of skewfoot as a deformity and it has typically been mentioned in conjunction with metatarsus adductus.

Napiontek[9] described four clinical types of skewfoot. The first is the congenital idiopathic type, which is characterized by supple deformities and very little rearfoot valgus. These deformities respond very well to conservative management. The second type is congenital and is associated with syndromes or systemic disorders. Among this group there is a high correlation with diastrophic dwarfism and skewfoot.[10]

[a] Highline Foot & Ankle Clinic, Franciscan Medical Group, 16233 Sylvester Road. SW G-10, Seattle, WA 98166, USA
[b] Franciscan Foot & Ankle Institute, Saint Francis Hospital, 34509 9th Avenue South Suite 306, Federal Way, WA 98003, USA
[c] Northwest Podiatric Foundation, 7315 212th Street SW Suite 103, Edmonds, Seattle, WA 98026, USA
* Corresponding author. Highline Foot & Ankle Clinic, Franciscan Medical Group, 16233 Sylvester Road. SW G-10, Seattle, WA 98166.
E-mail address: byronhutchinson@fhshealth.org

Clin Podiatr Med Surg 27 (2010) 93–104
doi:10.1016/j.cpm.2009.09.005
0891-8422/09/$ – see front matter © 2010 Elsevier Inc. All rights reserved.

podiatric.theclinics.com

Osteogenesis imperfecta and skewfoot has also been reported.[11] Neurogenic skew-foot is the third type and may exist in any of the major childhood neurogenic disorders. The fourth type is iatrogenic skewfoot, resulting from inappropriate casting or surgical intervention in children with talipes equinovarus.

There has been an increased awareness of this skewfoot in the past 20 years, but specific guidelines regarding treatment have not been established.[12] Jawish and colleagues[13] reported on 55 skewfeet in 31 children and determined that the valgus of the heel was transitory and secondary to forefoot rigidity. The majority of their patients did well with conservative treatment or surgical treatment focused at the correction of the metatarsus adductus. Mosca[14] reported on 31 severe, symptomatic valgus deformities of the rearfoot in 20 children who had flatfoot or skewfoot that were corrected by Evans calcaneal osteotomy. Twenty-six of the patients had an underlying neuromuscular disorder, which represents the most severe forms of skewfoot. The majority of articles discuss surgical treatment after conservative care has failed to correct the deformity with little mention of the severity of the symptomatology or what effect the deformity has on recreational activities or activities of daily living.[8] It is the opinion of this author that the establishment of the effects of the residual deformity on performance at a specific age is much more important than whether the deformity has not been completely corrected following conservative manage-ment—especially in those types of skewfoot previously outlined that are not rigid or do not involve neuromuscular disorders. Treating radiographic findings or parental concerns without considering the child's symptoms is a harbinger for poor outcomes.

CLINICAL EVALUATION

Skewfoot typically presents with peritalar subluxation in conjunction with metatarsus adductus. The calcaneus, cuboid, and navicular are all rotated laterally beneath the talus and the navicular articulates on the lateral side of the talar head resulting in a adducted forefoot, normal midfoot, and hindfoot valgus (**Fig. 1**).[6] The position of the forefoot may be deviated in several planes. Simple metatarsus adductus will be characterized by deviation of the metatarsals at Lisfranc joint in the transverse plane (**Fig. 2**). More complex forms may present in multiple planes. Identification of the complexity of the metatarsus adductus will help the physician determine the appropriate conservative or surgical treatment.

Appreciation of the resting attitude of the foot is important. Looking from the plantar aspect of the foot, is the rearfoot neutral and the forefoot deviated or is there a rearfoot

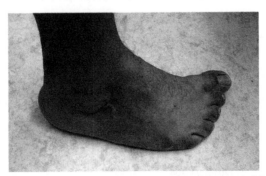

Fig. 1. Lateral view of a typical skewfoot. (Note that the heel is slightly lifted off the ground, which is secondary to concomitant equinus.)

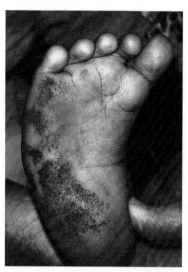

Fig. 2. Plantar aspect of a child with a simple metatarsus adductus deformity. Here the rear-foot is rectus.

deformity? Assessment of the weight-bearing attitude of the foot can assist the practitioner in the evaluation of deformity compensation. Mild deformities may become more severe with weight bearing and it is important to assess the dynamic nature of the deformity by simulating weight bearing.

The compensation can become more pronounced with weight bearing and failure to recognize this can dramatically affect treatment (**Fig. 3**). One must determine whether the deformity is rigid or flexible in regard to both the forefoot and rearfoot. A flexible deformity will probably respond to conservative therapy if initiated in a timely fashion (**Fig. 4**). Typically, patients under 3 years old have a flexible or semiflexible metatarsus

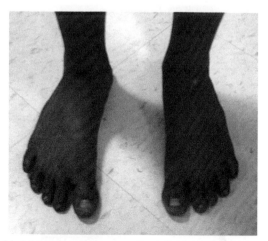

Fig. 3. A 12-year-old child with a flatfoot on the left and a skewfoot on the right. In this skewfoot, notice the compensation in the rearfoot and the accentuation of the metatarsus adductus.

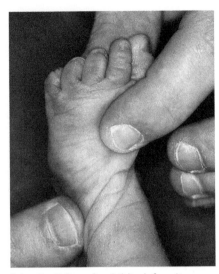

Fig. 4. Demonstration of the flexibility of a child's deformity.

adductus. Patients over 4 years old tend to develop a progressively more rigid deformity.[5]

Torsional abnormalities need to be considered in patients with metatarsus adductus. Deformities in the rearfoot or torsional abnormalities in the lower extremity can produce a "normal" looking foot. Assessment of hip and knee range of motion should be a standard part of the examination. Developmental hip dysplasia has been reported as more common in metatarsus adductus.[15] Torsional abnormalities of the tibia and femur have been identified with metatarsus adductus as well.[16] Therefore, the examiner should assess the existence of torsional abnormalities with the appropriate examination (**Fig. 5**).

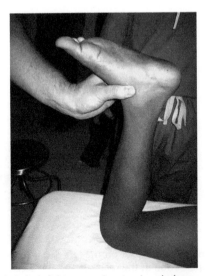

Fig. 5. The thigh-foot axis is helpful in assessing torsional abnormalities.

In older children, skewfoot deformity may be associated with juvenile hallux valgus and postural symptoms related to their flatfoot deformity. Placing the subtalar joint in the neutral position will readily reveal the metatarsus adductus or accentuate the juvenile hallux valgus deformity.

RADIOGRAPHIC EVALUATION

Several investigators, including this author, feel that radiographs are not imperative to evaluate or prognosticate metatarsus adductus.[17] Accurate measurements are difficult to reproduce.[18] In addition, the age and flexibility of the deformity are better prognosticating factors than radiographic findings. However, radiographic assessment may help to confirm the presence of complex deformities or the presence of rearfoot compensation and should still be obtained.

There are numerous methods described for the radiographic assessment of metatarsus adductus in the fully ossified skeleton.[19–24] In the infant or toddler foot, these measurements are difficult to recreate with accuracy because of the lack of ossification. Ganley and Ganley[25] have described a technique of measurement that the author prefers to use in these situations. They described using the talus and calcaneus as points of reference relative to the metatarsals in determining the existence of metatarsus adductus.

The measurement of Kyte's talocalcaneal angle is usually 20 to 25 degrees and any rearfoot component can be excluded with this measurement (**Fig. 6**). The calcaneal second metatarsal angle is usually 15 plus or minus 3 degrees.[25] If metatarsus adductus exists, it can be determined by subtracting 15 degrees from this angular measurement (**Fig. 7**). The lateral radiograph may demonstrate the degree of compensation in the rearfoot. The existence of significant pronation in the rearfoot will be seen as an anterior break in the cyma line and a talar bisection below the bisection of the first metatarsal. The lateral talocalcaneal angle will be above 45 degrees and the calcaneal inclination angle will be decreased.

In the ossified skeleton, the traditional method used for measuring metatarsus adductus has been to measure the lesser tarsus axis with the longitudinal axis of

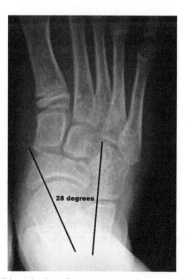

Fig. 6. Radiograph of a child with skewfoot. Normal Kyte's angle is 20–25 degrees.

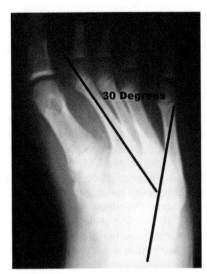

Fig. 7. Radiograph of metatarsus adductus in the underdeveloped skeleton of a child using the calcaneal-second metatarsal angle. This measurement is obtained by measuring the angle, in this case 45 degrees, and subtracting the normal angle of 15 degrees, giving the absolute value of 30 degrees in this example.

the metatarsals.[26] There has been controversy about the actual measurement, but this author considers anything over 20 degrees to be significant.[27–30] Taking radiographs in the rearfoot neutral position can also give the examiner valuable information regarding the amount of metatarsus adductus present and how it is compensated for in the rearfoot. The presence of a juvenile hallux valgus deformity can also be evaluated with this maneuver, which can help in surgical planning. Obtaining ankle films is also important to rule out a ball and socket ankle joint or other ankle pathology.

Other diagnostic methods have been established in the evaluation of metatarsus adductus and skewfoot, including photography and MRI. The author has not found any of these methods useful in either evaluation or prognosticating response to treatment.[31–33]

TREATMENT

Agnew[34] summarized treatment very effectively when he said, "In the absence of a reliable prognostic indicator or test, the decision whether to treat and how to treat a patient with metatarsus adductus remains more of an art than a science." There are no outcome-based studies on the treatment of metatarsus adductus and many recommendations are made based on individual experience or small series articles. Recommending observation in hopes of spontaneous resolution is not an effective method of treatment. Every practitioner sees uncorrected cases of metatarsus adductus and skewfoot at different stages and ages that need treatment because of symptoms related to the residual deformity, but no one really knows what percentage this represents in the overall incidence of metatarsus adductus or skewfoot. Not all patients that have metatarsus adductus in their adult lives have problems with the deformity.

There are numerous articles that speak to the success of decreasing the deformity at a young age and in a flexible foot.[35–38] Very few would argue that early treatment is safer and easier than treatment that is delayed. This establishes the basis for initial treatment of this deformity. Initial treatment should begin as soon as possible and involves manipulation and casting. Eventually these patients undergo splinting and shoe therapy. In those patients where there is concern about the development of a skewfoot, orthotic control is paramount.

Surgical intervention has been employed at all ages in the treatment of metatarsus adductus and skewfoot based in part on the failure of conservative therapy to resolve the deformity.[7,12–14,34–41] Soft tissue procedures have been performed as early as 2 years of age and as late as 7 to 8 years of age because of residual deformity.[35–38,42–44] The author's experience with Heyman, Herndon, and Strong procedures has generally been favorable; however, it is difficult to determine if a child at 2 years of age has symptoms as a result of the deformity or if the deformity will cause problems in the future. Therefore, it is important to consider surgical intervention in this age range only when there is significant deformity present and there are underlying neuromuscular reasons to operate. It has been the author's experience that soft tissue procedures can have a significantly high recurrence. An increase in the radiographic appearance of the metatarsus adductus and failure of conservative care is not enough to embark on a surgical misadventure in these patients.

Consideration of a family history of a similar deformity and how this deformity has affected those individuals should be of paramount concern to the clinician recommending surgery. Additionally, in children between ages 4 and 10 (before skeletal maturity) the surgeon should mainly consider surgery if the deformity truly does effects the child's ability to walk and function. The vast majority of these young patients should not be treated surgically until they have hit skeletal maturity and the affects of the deformity can be determined based on their ability to function on a daily basis.

When surgery becomes necessary, there are a number of procedures that can be employed to improve the quality of life in individuals who have a skewfoot deformity. As discussed, the skewfoot deformity is the common long-term sequela of metatarsus adductus and typically the deformity is rigid or semirigid. Therefore, surgical management is aimed at osseous correction at the apex of the deformity. There is usually a rigid adductus deformity and a partially compensated or fully compensated flatfoot deformity present. Typically, a combination of surgical procedures is used based on the clinical and radiographic evaluation.

The rearfoot deformity is usually addressed first and a number of hindfoot realignment procedures can be considered. There is consensus that some form of equinus release needs to be done during the surgical management of patients with skewfoot. The author prefers a gastrocnemius recession from a limited medial approach in the vast majority of situations (**Fig. 8**). Rarely, the patient may need a tendoachilles lengthening. In the patients with neurogenic types of skewfoot, the tendoachilles lengthening is the preferred method for equinus release.

Mosca[14] reported results with a combination of an Evans osteotomy, percutaneous tendoachilles lengthening, and a medial cuneiform osteotomy in 21 patients. The equinus release was performed initially, followed by the calcaneal osteotomy. Any additional procedures were done after hindfoot alignment was achieved. This combination was performed in children with significant deformities, and results were very favorable. Benard[45] reported on a single case in a 9-year-old boy of multiple metatarsal osteotomies and a medial displacement calcaneal osteotomy. Rearfoot arthrodesis procedures can also be performed in selected situations where arthrosis is present, or in the face of a progressive neuromuscular deformity.

In addressing the midfoot and forefoot component of the deformity, there have been a number of surgical reports. Multiple metatarsal osteotomy techniques have been

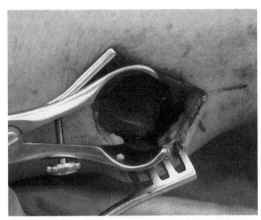

Fig. 8. Medial gastrocnemius recession. Using a nasal speculum, the fibers of the gastrocnemius are elevated off the soleus and sectioned from medial toward lateral with a nasal scissor, taking care to visualize the sural nerve before cutting the fibers.

outlined with subtle variations in technical performance.[7,39–41] Most reports of these techniques have been favorable and the decision of what technique to use is determined by surgeon preference.

Opening wedge medial cuneiform osteotomy was first proposed by Fowler and colleagues[46] in 1959 for the correction of a cavovarus deformity. In the late 1970s and early 1980s, the procedure became popular for treating residual varus deformity in talipes equinovarus.[47–49] The combination of this opening wedge medial cuneiform osteotomy and a closing wedge osteotomy of the cuboid has become very popular to address this component of the deformity.[50,51] Brink and Levitsky[30] prefer opening wedge osteotomy and cuboid closing wedge osteotomy to deal with the adductus, instead of multiple metatarsal osteotomies.

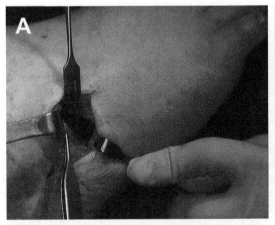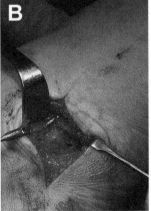

Fig. 9. Intraoperative photographs demonstrating closing wedge cuboid osteotomy. (*A*) The wedge of bone was removed before taking this photograph. Identification of the adjacent joints is imperative to plan the osteotomy equidistant from these two joint surfaces. (*B*) A single bone staple provides fixation of the closed cuboid osteotomy. Alternatively, use a smooth wire for fixation.

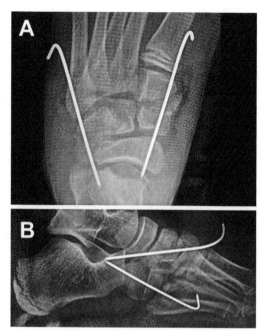

Fig. 10. Postoperative anterior-posterior radiograph (*A*) and lateral radiograph (*B*) of a cuboid and cuneiform osteotomy with wire fixation. (Note the effect of the procedure on the forefoot.)

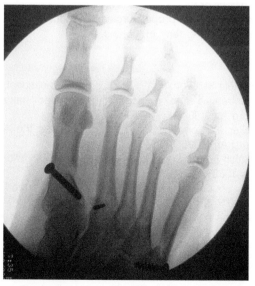

Fig. 11. Intraoperative fluoroscopic view of a modified Lepird procedure in an adolescent patient.

Napiontek and colleagues[52] reported on opening wedge osteotomy of the medial cuneiform in 25 children before the age of four. One child in this series had a skewfoot, and talipes equinovarus was the diagnosis in the majority of the other children. Before this report, there were no recommendations of performing medial cuneiform osteotomy in this age group because of concerns about the potential for nonunion of the bone graft.[17] Napiontek and colleagues[52] found that not only did the bone graft incorporate, but the two halves of the cuneiform grew independently and that overcorrection was a concern.

In severe cases of skewfoot, the author prefers the Evans calcaneal osteotomy for correction of the hindfoot component of the skewfoot. In mild-to-moderate cases, a medializing calcaneal osteotomy is also useful. The author has found that the forefoot deformity is more problematic than the rearfoot component. If the radiographic evaluation indicates that there is a mild-to-moderate adductus, it is the author's preference to perform a medial cuneiform opening osteotomy and a closing cuboid osteotomy (**Figs. 9** and **10**). If the deformity is severe, multiple metatarsal osteotomies may be needed to get the amount of correction necessary. There are various techniques for performing this; however, oblique closing wedge osteotomies of the first and fifth metatarsals and oblique lesser metatarsal osteotomies of the second to fourth in the frontal plane are the author's preference (**Fig. 11**). In rare cases, the abductor tendon is resected at the level of the first metatarsal phalangeal joint. If the patient has a progressive neuromuscular deformity, arthrodesis procedures are favored. Isolated subtalar joint fusions or medial column procedures are preferred. In cases with significant deformity or arthrosis, a triple arthrodesis may be unavoidable.

SUMMARY

Skewfoot is a rare condition that is often missed early in a child's development. Mild and flexible forms can be successfully treated with cast immobilization and shoe therapy. In more severe forms, surgical intervention is indicated if there are underlying neuromuscular conditions or the individual is affected on a daily basis because of the deformity. Careful evaluation and proper surgical procedures selection can realign the foot, resulting in favorable long-term outcomes.

REFERENCES

1. Farsetti P, Weinstein SL, Ponseti IV. The long-term functional and radiographic outcomes of untreated and non-operatively treated metatarsus adductus. J Bone Joint Surg Am 1994;76(2):257–65.
2. Ponsetti IV, Becker JR. Congenital metatarsus adductus: the results of treatment. J Bone Joint Surg Am 1996;48:702.
3. LaPorta G, Sokoloff H. Metatarsus adductus: a two-year follow up of 22 cases. Hershey update 1980;1.
4. Katz K, David R, Soudry M. Below-knee plaster cast for the treatment of metatarsus adductus. J Pediatr Orthop 1999;19(1):49–50.
5. Wan SC. Metatarsus adductus and skewfoot deformity. Clin Podiatr Med Surg 2006;23(1):23–40.
6. Berg EE. A reappraisal of metatarsus adductus and skewfoot. J Bone Joint Surg Am 1986;68(8):1185–96.
7. McCormick D, Blount WP. Metatarsus adducto varus. JAMA 1949;141:449.
8. Bleck EE. Metatarsus adductus: classification and relationship to outcomes of treatment. J Pediatr Orthop 1983;3(1):2–9.

9. Napiontek M. Skewfoot. J Pediatr Orthop 2002;22(1):130–3.
10. Ryoppy, Poussa S, Merkanto MJ, et al. Foot deformities in diastrophic dysplasia. J Bone Joint Surg Br 1992;74:441–4.
11. Mirzayan R, Cepkinian V, Yu J, et al. Skewfoot in patients with osteogenesis imperfecta. Foot Ankle Int 2000;2:768–71.
12. Peterson HA. Skewfoot (forefoot adduction with heel valgus). J Pediatr Orthop 1986;6(1):24–30.
13. Jawish R, Rigault P, Padovani JP, et al. [The Z-shaped or serpentine foot in children and adolescents]. Chir Pediatr 1990;31(6):314–21 [in French].
14. Mosca VS. Calcaneal lengthening for valgus deformity of the hindfoot. Results in children who had severe, symptomatic flatfoot and skewfoot. J Bone Joint Surg Am 1995;77(4):500–12.
15. Wynne-Davies R, Littlejohn A, Gormley J. Aetiology and interrelationship of some common skeleton deformities. J Med Genet 1982;19:321–8.
16. Kite HJ. Congenital metatarsus varus. J Bone Joint Surg Am 1967;49:388–97.
17. Thompson GH, Simmons GW. Congenital talipes equinovarus (clubfeet) and metatarsus adductus. In: Drennan JC, editor. The child's foot and ankle. New York: Raven Press; 1992. p. 146–58.
18. Hlavac HF. Differences in x-ray findings with varied positioning of the foot. J Am Podiatry Assoc 1967;57:465–71.
19. Brown J, Purvis DG, Kaplan EG, et al. Berman-Gartland operation for correction of resistant adduction of the forefoot of the foot. J Am Podiatry Assoc 1977;67:841.
20. Engel E, Erlich N, Krems I. A simplified metatarsus adductus angle. J Am Podiatry Assoc 1983;73:620.
21. Fliegel O. Congenital pes adductus. Bull Hosp Joint Dis 1955;16:65.
22. Schoenhaus H, Rotman S, Meshon A. A review of normal intermetatarsal angles. J Am Podiatry Assoc 1973;63:88.
23. Gamble FO, Yale I. Clinical root roentgenology. Huntington (NY): Krieger; 1975. p. 284.
24. Bankart B. Metatarsus varus. Br Med J 1921;2:685.
25. Ganley JV, Ganley TJ. Metatarsus adductus deformity. In: McGlamry ED, Banks AS, Downey MS, editors. Comprehensive textbook of foot surgery. 2nd edition. Baltimore (MD): Williams & Wilkins; 1992. p. 829–52.
26. Root ML, Orien WP, Weed JH, et al. Biomechanical examinations of the foot. Los Angeles (CA): Clinical Biomechanics; 1971. p. 33.
27. Yu GV, DiNapoli DR. Surgical management of hallux abductovalgus with concomitant metararsus adductus. In: McGlamry ED, editor. Reconstructive surgery of the foot and leg: update '89. Tucker (GA): Podiatry Institute; 1989. p. 262–8.
28. Weissman SD. Biomechanically acquired foot types. In: Weissman SD, editor. Radiology of the foot. Baltimore (MD): Williams & Wilkins; 1983. p. 50–76.
29. Heatherington VJ, Lehtinen J, Grill F. The pediatric patient. In: Levy LA, Heatherington VJ, editors. Principles and practice of podiatric medicine. New York: Churchill Lifingstone; 1990. p. 571–612.
30. Brink DS, Levitsky DR. Cuneiform and cuboid wedge osteotomies for correction of residual metatarsus adductus: a surgical review. J Foot Ankle Surg 1995;34(4):371–8.
31. Smith JT, Bleck EE, Gamble JG, et al. Simple method of documenting metatarsus adductus. J Pediatr Orthop 1991;11(5):679–80.
32. Hubbard AM, Davidson RS, Meyer JS, et al. Magnetic resonance imaging of skewfoot. J Bone Joint Surg Am 1996;78(3):389–97.

33. Wenger DR, Rang M. The art and practice of children's orthopedics. New York: Raven Press; 1993.
34. Agnew PS. Metatarsus adductus and allied disorders. In: McGlamry ED, Banks AS, Downey MS, et al, editors. Comprehensive textbook of foot and ankle surgery. 3rd edition. Baltimore (MD): Williams & Wilkins; 2001. p. 915–42.
35. Heyman CH, Herndon CH, Strong JM. Mobilization of the tarsometatarsal and intermetatarsal joints for the correction of resistant adduction of the forepart of the foot in congenital clubfoot or congenital metatarsus varus. J Bone Joint Surg Am 1958;40:299.
36. Stark JG, Johanson JE, Winter RB, et al. The Heyman-Herndon tarsometatarsal capsulotomy for metatarsus adductus: results in 48 feet. J Pediatr Orthop 1987;7:305–10.
37. Johnson JB. A preliminary report on chondrotomies: a new surgical approach to metatarsus adductus in children. J Am Podiatry Assoc 1978;68(12):808–13.
38. Sgarlato TE. A discussion of metatarsus adductus. Arch Podiatr Med Foot Surg 1973;1:35.
39. Berman A, Gartland JJ. Metatarsal osteotomyfor the correction of adduction of the fore part of the foot in children. J Bone Joint Surg Am 1971;53:498.
40. Steytler JCS, Van Der Walt ID. Correction of resistant adduction of the forefoot in congenital club foot and congenital metatarsus varus by metatarsal osteotomy. Br J Surg 1966;53:558.
41. Yu GV, Johng B, Freireich R. Surgical management of metatarsus adductus deformity. Clin Podiatr Med Surg 1987;4:207–32.
42. Mitchel GP. Adductor hallucis release in congenital metatarsus varus. Int Orthop 1980;3:299–304.
43. Thomson SA. Hallux varus and metatarsus varus: a five-year study (1954–1958). Clin Orthop 1960;16:109–18.
44. Lichtblau S. Section of the adductor hallucis tendon for correction of metatarsus adductus varus deformity. Clin Orthop 1975;110:227–32.
45. Benard MA. Treatment of skewfoot by multiple lesser tarsal osteotomie and calcaneal osteotomy. J Foot Surg 1980;29(5):504–9.
46. Fowler SB, Brooks AL, Parrish TF. The cavovarus foot. J Bone Joint Surg Am 1959;41:757.
47. Johanning K. Exocochleatio ossis cuboidie in the treatment of pes equino varus. Acta Orthop Scand 1958;27:310.
48. Hoffman AA, Constine RN, McBridge GG, et al. Osteotomy of the first cuneiform as treatment of residual adduction of the forepart of the foot in clubfoot. J Bone Joint Surg Am 1984;66:985.
49. Lareaux RL, Hosey T. Results of surgical treatment of talipes equino valgus by means of navicular-cuneiform arthrodesis with midcuboid osteotomy. J Foot Surg 1987;26:412–8.
50. Mosca VS. Skewfoot deformity in children: correction by calcaneal neck lengthening and medial cuneiform opening wedge osteotomies. J Pediatr Orthop 1993;13:807.
51. Harley BD, Fritzhand AJ, Little JM, et al. Abductory midfoot osteotomy procedure for metatarsus adductus. J Foot Ankle Surg 1995;34:153–62.
52. Napiontek M, Tomasz K, Marek T. Opening wedge osteotomy of the medial cuneiform before age 4 years in the treatment of forefoot adduction. J Pediatr Orthop 2003;23:65–9.

Tarsal Coalitions: Etiology, Diagnosis, Imaging, and Stigmata

Klaus J. Kernbach, DPM

KEYWORDS

- Tarsal coalition • Pes planus
- Middle facet talocalcaneal coalition
- Calcaneal fibular remodeling
- Calcaneonavicular coalition • Flatfoot

Tarsal coalition is a congenital condition characterized by the aberrant union (osseous or fibrous) between 2 bones in the rearfoot, most commonly talocalcaneal coalition (TCC), calcaneonavicular coalition (CNC), and talonavicular coalition (TNC), that results in restriction or absence of motion. Cruveilhier[1] in 1829 and Zuckerlandl[2] in 1877, documented the anatomic descriptions of tarsal coalition. Harris and Beath,[3] in their landmark article (1948), popularized the association between tarsal coalition and peroneal spastic flatfoot. Since then, associations between tarsal coalition and a variety of coexisting conditions have been reported. These associations are believed to be secondary effects of the coalition and/or fixed rearfoot position, such as pes planovalgus (also known as coalition-associated flatfoot), equinus, rearfoot arthrosis, traction spurring of the talonavicular and calcaneonavicular joint, ball-and-socket ankle joint, and/or calcaneal fibular remodeling (CFR).[4–19]

INCIDENCE AND ETIOLOGY

The incidence of tarsal coalition has been estimated to be between 2% and 13%.[20–23] Without the use of advanced imaging, most studies have estimated the incidence to be less than 2%.[3,23] Pfitzner's[20] cadaveric study from 1896 and more recent literature have suggested that tarsal coalition is more common than classically described.[21,22] In a 1984 review article on tarsal coalitions and peroneal spastic flatfoot, Mosier and Asher[11] commented that Pfitzner's cadaveric dissection of 520 feet of skeletons may represent "the most accurate incidence study of tarsal coalition in the general population." Evaluating for TCC and CNC, Pfitzner[20] identified an incidence of almost 6%. Solomon and colleagues,[22] in their dissection and computed tomography (CT) review of 100 cadaveric feet, estimated the incidence of tarsal coalition to be nearly 13%. In

Financial disclosures, none; Conflicts of interest, none.
Department of Podiatry, Kaiser Foundation Hospital, 975 Sereno Drive, Vallejo, CA 94589, USA
E-mail address: kkernbach@gmail.com

2008, a prospective evaluation of 667 consecutive ankle magnetic resonance imaging (MRI) scans has suggested that the frequency of tarsal coalitions may be as high as 11%, although there may be population bias in this particular study.[21] Stormont and Peterson[23] authored one of the most frequently cited articles on the relative incidence of tarsal coalition. In their review of the literature spanning almost 60 years, they found that TCC and CNC are the most common locations of coalition, with an incidence rate of 48.1% and 43.6%, respectively. It is clear that more incidence-based studies that use advanced imaging would be useful in better understanding how frequently tarsal coalitions occur.

Bilateral tarsal coalition is not uncommon. Leonard[19] identified the presence of bilateral coalition at 80% in his review of 31 patients and 98 of their first-degree relatives. Stormont and Peterson[23] estimated the incidence of bilateral TCC and CNC to be about 22% and 68%, respectively. Solomon and colleagues[22] found the incidence of bilateral coalition to be as high as 40% in their cadaveric dissection. Lahey and colleagues[24] identified bilateral involvement in more than half of the TCCs and TNCs in their series.

The exact cause of tarsal coalition is not entirely clear, but it seems to be a condition that one is born with. Histopathologic studies have identified the presence of coalition in embryonic development[25] and immediately after birth on surgical dissection.[23] Failure of embryonic mesenchyme has been implicated as a potential cause of tarsal coalition, and it has been theorized to present as an autosomal dominant trait with variable penetrance.[19,25,26] Leonard[19] also suggests a nonspecific expression of the involved gene whereby coalition phenotype is not consistent along the familial lineage. Various syndromes and conditions have identified the presence of tarsal coalitions. They include Nievergelt syndrome, carpal coalition, symphalangism, phocomelia, fibular hemimelia, and other gross limb anomalies.[19,27–30] There does not appear to be a correlation between tarsal coalition and accessory tarsal bones.[22]

It has been suggested that the incidence of tarsal coalitions is nearly equal between men and women, although some studies do identify a male prevalence.[19,23,31,32] Conway and Cowell[31] reported 4 times as many men with tarsal coalition than women in their retrospective review. In a large epidemiologic review of nearly 1 million foot and ankle surgical procedures performed in Australia over a 10-year period, Menz and colleagues[32] identified that men had 1.5 more surgeries for tarsal coalition than women. Stormont and Peterson[23] did not find a statistically significant difference in sex distribution.

DIAGNOSIS

Diagnosis of tarsal coalition is, first and foremost, a radiographic inclusion diagnosis. The history identifies symptoms and behavior patterns that seem to occur as a result of a symptomatic coalition. The patient and family members may describe a lack of physical activity with peers and siblings. Parents may acknowledge a family history of similar foot problems and/or whether their child is more sedentary because of the complaints of foot fatigue or pain. There may be a noticeable limp or a reluctance to run. In some cases, the symptoms of tarsal coalition may be unmasked (and/or initiated) by a history of trauma, such as an ankle sprain.[11,13,16] The pain is frequently exacerbated with activity and alleviated with rest. When coalition-associated flatfoot is present, patients may identify the flatfoot as being the pathologic problem and the cause for the pain.[8] Unexplained hindfoot pain with or without peroneal spasms may be identified.[11,15] Less commonly, tarsal tunnel syndrome–like symptoms may also be present.[15]

Typically, the symptoms associated with tarsal coalition occur in puberty or adolescence.[23] CNC usually manifests with symptoms at an earlier age than TCC.[11,23,24] Some investigators have suggested that symptoms coincide with the ossification of the tarsal coalition, as reported by Jayakumar and Cowell,[4] between the ages of 8 and 12 years and 12 and 16 years for CNC and TCC, respectively.[11,23] Lahey and colleagues[24] identified that ossification of the TNC has little, if any, relationship to the onset of clinical symptoms.

Tarsal coalitions may present in conjunction with a rigid flatfoot. In severe cases, the flatfoot itself alerts the physician to suspect a tarsal coalition. Obviously, a rigid foot is highly suspicious. The inability of the rearfoot to supinate while performing a single leg toe rise should suggest the presence of coalition to the practitioner. Salomão and colleagues[13] also refer to this "tip toe test." The test helps to differentiate the flexible flatfeet from the rigid. If there is pain while performing the "tip toe test," the posterior tibialis tendon should be palpated and evaluated as a potential area of additional pathology.[8]

On physical examination, CNC may manifest with tenderness to palpation just distal to the lateral malleolus and sinus tarsi at the calcaneonavicular interval.[11] Similarly, TCC may manifest with pain in the medial rearfoot at the sustentaculum tali, just inferior to the medial malleolus.[11] With TCC it is also not uncommon to find an increased girth to the hindfoot at the sustentaculum tali, just inferior to the medial malleolus. When there is a flatfoot deformity, whether flexible or rigid, it is also not uncommon to have lateral symptoms related to subfibular and/or lateral talar process impingement pain.[15,17,33,34] Some refer to this malady as sinus tarsi syndrome, and it can be found concomitantly with and without tarsal coalition.[15,33]

Rigid pediatric flatfoot commonly occurs as a result of a tarsal coalition,[3,13,15,33] and many investigators have identified that the symptoms associated with tarsal coalition may be exacerbated with the severity of the flatfoot deformity.[8–11,35,36] With symptomatic tarsal coalition, concomitant ankle equinus, posterior tibialis tendon dysfunction, CFR, and/or other segmental pedal misalignment with or without degenerative arthrosis may be present and can be identified on advanced imaging.[8,9,17,37,38]

IMAGING

Tarsal coalitions are often identified on simple radiographic examinations. In evaluating for different types of coalition, radiographs should include weight-bearing anteroposterior (AP), medial oblique (MO), and lateral projections.[12,13,33,39] CNCs are best identified on the MO view (**Fig. 1**). TNCs are visible on the lateral and AP foot views, and physicians may overlook the coalition and misrepresent the talar head as simply being enlarged (**Fig. 2**). Although TCCs may be identified on lateral view, they are well visualized with a Harris-Beath series (**Fig. 3**).[3,12,13] This "modified calcaneal axial view" at 45°, whereby the knees are flexed and the tibiotalar joint is dorsiflexed to prevent radiographic superimposition of the leg over the sustentaculum tali, will demonstrate obliquity present at the middle facet relative to the posterior facet of the subtalar joint, which is often diagnostic for TCC.[3] Plain films should also be scrutinized for other radiographic features that are common to tarsal coalition, including the presence of rearfoot arthrosis, dorsal talar beaking,[3,15,21,40,41] blunted lateral talar process,[40] "anteater nose" sign,[21,42] reverse anteater sign,[21] C sign,[15,40] drunken waiter sign,[21] a ball-and-socket ankle joint,[15,43] an absent middle facet sign,[40] dysmorphic talus, and/or sustentaculum tali.[21,40] The radiographic C sign, (**Fig. 4**) identified on lateral weight-bearing plain films, is sensitive and specific for the diagnosis of

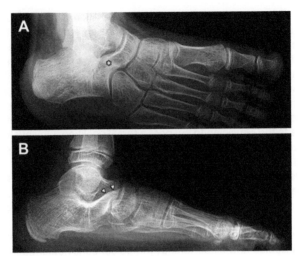

Fig. 1. Complete osseous coalition CNC (*asterisk*) best visualized on MO view (*A*), and "anteater sign" (*arrow heads*) seen on lateral view (*B*).

TCC, at least in 1 study.[16] Other investigators have suggested that the C sign may be more specific for flatfoot than for TCC.[18]

Advanced imaging, such as CT and MRI, is useful in the diagnostic evaluation of the associated stigmata of coalitions and in surgical planning.[8,9,15–17,21,33,37,40,44–50] Both CT and MRI are useful; however, CT has been regarded as the best method of diagnostic imaging for coalition and to distinguish between osseous and fibrous coalitions (**Fig. 5**).[16,33,45] In a detailed analysis of CNC using multiplanar three-dimensional CT, CT was identified as the gold standard in identifying coalition.[33] However, it has been suggested that CT scans may have a low sensitivity for detecting nonosseous tarsal coalition.[22] Other investigators have advocated MRI over CT,[21] and MRI may help evaluate concomitant tendon pathology and/or marrow edema in certain circumstances (**Fig. 6**). One should evaluate the size of the coalition and whether or not the coalition is fibrous or osseous.[33,45] Rassi and colleagues[51] have suggested that technetium-99m bone scans be used for the evaluation of arthrofibrosis involving the middle facet of the talocalcaneal joint in children and adolescents when other diagnostic imaging results are inconclusive.

TARSAL COALITION STIGMATA
Coalition Concomitant Pes Planus

The association between tarsal coalition and the pediatric pes planovalgus deformity has been well documented and is a common problem (**Fig. 7**),[4–19] although the incidence of flatfoot occurring within tarsal coalition is unclear. At least clinically, TCC seems to be most commonly associated with more severe flatfoot. CNC and TNC are less commonly associated with significant flatfoot deformity. The planus nature of the foot is not always considered a pathologic problem within the literature.[8,52] This is evident because many studies have focused on simple coalition resection and interpositional material rather than on the surgical management of the pedal misalignment.[13,53–57] With regard to TCC, poorer outcomes with simple resections

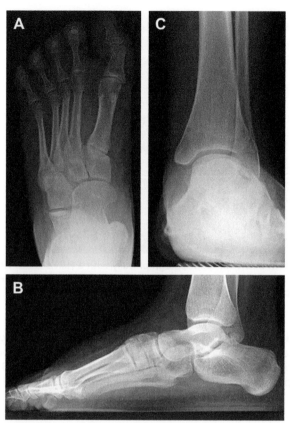

Fig. 2. Complete TNC on the (*A*) anteroposterior and (*B*) lateral weight-bearing views. Over time, a ball-and-socket ankle joint may develop (*C*) to compensate for the lack of motion ordinarily provided by the essential talonavicular joint. (*Courtesy of* Neal M. Blitz, DPM, Bronx, New York, NY.)

and preoperative heel valgus have led surgeons to consider the pathologic nature of the concomitant flatfoot.[5,9] Surgeons now address the pes planus problem primarily and perform flatfoot reconstructions.[5,8–10,38,58]

Peroneal Spasm

Harris and Beath[3] popularized the association between tarsal coalition, rigid flatfoot deformity, and peroneal tendon spasm. Although, they themselves observe that "the term peroneal spastic flatfoot is often applied indiscriminately and inaccurately to certain rigid flat feet which arise from quite different causes."[3] They theorized that with TCC and CNC, the peroneal tendons adaptively shorten in response to the rigid valgus deformity,[3] although peroneal lengthenings are not generally performed after coalition resection.

CFR

CFR is a newly described entity, in which fixed valgus abutment of the calcaneus against the fibula may result in a morphologic degenerative process between the 2 segments.[17] Features of CFR include pseudoarticulation, spurring, and cystic

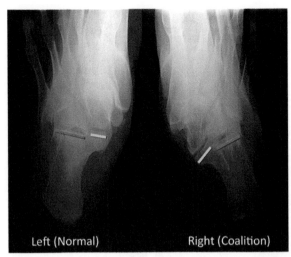

Fig. 3. A TCC is often best visualized radiographically with a Harris-Beath view. In the presence of a coalition (*right foot*), the middle facet (*blue line*) is oriented obliquely to the posterior facet (*orange line*).

changes (see **Fig. 7**C). Although these radiographic changes occur and appear pathologic, it is unclear if this entity is part of the pain cascade. CFR has been evaluated as an additional area of pathology in coalition associated with flatfoot.[17] Spurring, cysts, and other morphologic changes have been identified with CFR, and this suggests

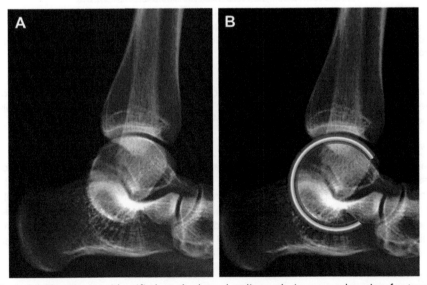

Fig. 4. (*A*) The "C" sign, identified on the lateral radiograph, is a secondary sign for tarsal coalition. The "C" represents the articular curvature of the talar body and the sustentaculum tali bound together by the middle facet talocalcalcaneal coalition. (*B*) The "C" is attenuated in this image.

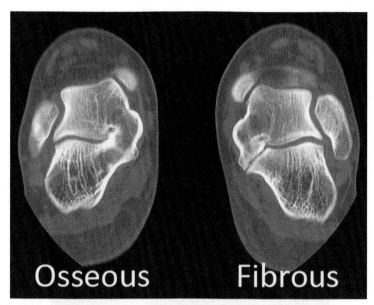

Fig. 5. Bilateral middle facet tarsal coalition, osseous and fibrous, best visualized on coronal CT. (*Courtesy of* Neal M. Blitz, DPM, Bronx, New York.)

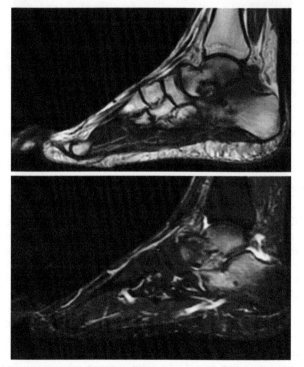

Fig. 6. Matched MRI T1-weighted (*top*) and T2-weighted (*bottom*) sagittal images depicting extensive marrow edema of the talus and calcaneus in a 17-year-old boy with symptomatic peroneal spasm, pes planovalgus deformity, and subtle calcaneonavicular bar. Also note the suggestive talar beaking best depicted on the T1-image.

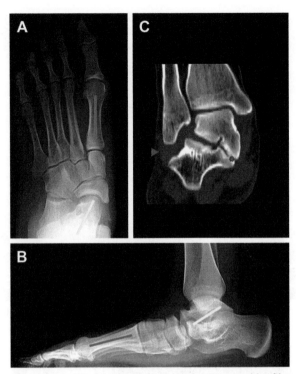

Fig. 7. (*A, B*) Symptomatic coalition concomitant pes planus caused by fibrous middle facet tarsal coalition in a 14-year-old girl. Weight-bearing radiographs illustrate dorsilateral peritalar subluxation, dorsal talar beaking, hypoplastic talus, low calcaneal pitch, and high cuboid abduction angle. (*C*) Coronal CT best visualizes fibrous middle facet tarsal coalition (*purple asterisk*) and calcaneofibular remodeling (*red arrowhead*).

another potential pathologic degenerative process that may be associated with tarsal coalition in the setting of calcaneal valgus deformity.

Subtalar Joint Arthrosis

Arthrosis of the subtalar joint has long been associated with tarsal coalition, mainly middle facet TCC.[8,37,59,60] It is unclear why the posterior facet undergoes a degenerative process, and it is likely that the cause is multifactorial. The subtalar joint is 3-faceted and when coalition affects the middle facet, it is not unreasonable that a degenerative process would continue throughout the entire subtalar joint. Studies comparing the incidence of posterior facet arthrosis associated with TNC, CNC, and TCC would be interesting and useful.

Elsewhere in this issue, a staging system that allows physicians to grade the extent of arthrosis is presented by Blitz and Kernbach.[37] The extent of posterior facet arthrosis is graded as normal or mild arthrosis (stage I), moderate (stage II), and severe (stage III). Researchers have suggested that the type of coalition (osseous vs fibrous) may be associated with the extent of posterior facet arthrosis.[37] The presence of symptomatic arthrosis is critical in the workup of tarsal coalition because a degenerated joint may preclude simple coalition resection (with or without concomitant flatfoot reconstruction) and may require rearfoot fusion.[8,52]

Talar Beaking

Numerous investigators have identified that isolated talar beaking is not always characteristic of degeneration in the hindfoot joints (**Fig. 8**). The presence of talar beaking does not preclude coalition resection. Lemley and colleagues,[60] in their concise review of tarsal coalition, identified that "talar beaking is not a sign of arthrosis, and is not a contraindication to talocalcaneal coalition excision...." Swiontkowski and colleagues[41] identified that the talar beak "is not necessarily a degenerative spur, but rather a traction process occurring secondary to increased motion." The restriction of motion that is caused by the coalition, and in some instances the ankle joint equinus, contributes to this talar beaking because the essential talonavicular joint is forced to compensate for the lack of motion in the adjacent essential joints. Wilde and colleagues[9] found no association between talar beaking and surgical outcome. Kitaoka and colleagues[55] found that 5 of 6 patients with talar beaking had excellent results after isolated coalition resection.

Equinus

Equinus has long been associated with flatfoot, although its prevalence with tarsal coalition has not been specifically evaluated.[8,14,38,61] Studies do not exist that compare the presence of equinus amongst the various types of tarsal coalitions. Fixed valgus of the heel may perpetuate the equinus. Nonetheless, equinus correction often is performed in conjunction with coalition resections, and especially as part of a concomitant flatfoot reconstruction.[8,61] Kernbach and colleagues[8] performed equinus correction on all 6 feet that underwent single-stage flatfoot reconstruction with coalition resection. Yen and colleagues[38] have also acknowledged the contribution of the Achilles tendon to coalition-associated calcaneal valgus. Westberry and colleagues[14] have recognized unaddressed equinus as a contributing factor in failed isolated coalition resections and secondarily performed equinus correction when indicated.

Ball-and-Socket Ankle Joint

In some instances of tarsal coalition and/or congenital shortening of the lower extremity, a ball-and-socket ankle joint may develop (see **Fig. 2**B). A ball-and-socket ankle is an aberrant configuration of the tibiotalar joint, characterized by increased

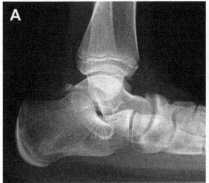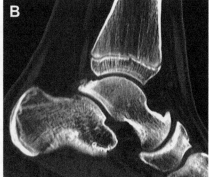

Fig. 8. A 13-year-old boy with symptomatic middle facet TCC. The middle facet coalition is not visualized; however, the dorsal talar beaking is depicted on radiography (A) and CT (B). Note that there is no significant talonavicular joint arthrosis.

tibial plafond and fibular concavity coupled with increased talar dome convexity. When associated with tarsal coalition, it is frequently an adaptive deformation to compensate for decreased inversion and eversion at the adjacent joints in the tritarsal complex. Pappas and Miller[43] have also suggested that the ball-and-socket ankle joint may be associated with an atavistic regression similar to the phenotype of the arboreal gorilla and/or a congenital syndrome of the lower extremity. Symptoms associated with the ball-and-socket ankle joint are typically rare, and preservation of the essential hindfoot and ankle joints should be a priority whenever possible.[8,59,62–67]

SUMMARY

The association between tarsal coalition and a variety of coexisting conditions has been reported over the past 60 years and continues to be better understood. These coexisting conditions (the stigmata of tarsal coalition) have been believed to be secondary effects of the coalition and/or fixed rearfoot position. They include pes planovalgus (also known as coalition-associated flatfoot), equinus, rearfoot arthrosis, traction spurring of the talonavicular and calcaneonavicular joint, ball-and-socket ankle joint, and/or CFR. Advanced imaging has provided significant insights into the concomitant pathology and understanding that the symptoms associated with tarsal coalition can be present for a myriad of different reasons. One should consider all the stigmata of tarsal coalition when considering a surgical reconstruction.

REFERENCES

1. Cruveilhier J. Anatomie pathologique du corps humain [Pathologic anatomy of the human corps]. Paris: Tome I.J.B. Bailliere; 1829 [in French].
2. Zuckerlandl E. Ueber einen Fall von Synostose zwischen Talus und Calcaneus [The synostosis between the talus and calcaneus]. Allg Wein Med Zeitung 1877;22:293–4 [in German].
3. Harris RI, Beath T. Etiology of peroneal spastic flat foot. J Bone Joint Surg Am 1948;30-B:624–34.
4. Jayakumar S, Cowell HR. Rigid flatfoot. Clin Orthop 1977;122:77–84.
5. Luhmann SJ, Schoenecker PL. Symptomatic talocalcaneal coalition resection: indications and results. J Pediatr Orthop 1998;18(6):748–54.
6. Rouvreau P, Pouliquen JC, Langlais J, et al. [Synostosis and tarsal coalitions in children. A study of 68 cases in 47 patients]. Rev Chir Orthop Reparatrice Appar Mot 1994;80(3):252–60 [in French].
7. Mosca VS. Calcaneal lengthening for valgus deformity of the hindfoot. Results in children who had severe, symptomatic flatfoot and skewfoot. J Bone Joint Surg Am 1995;77(4):500–12.
8. Kernbach KJ, Blitz NM, Rush SM. Bilateral single stage middle facet coalition resection combined with flatfoot reconstruction. A report of 3 cases and review of the literature. Investigations involving middle facet coalitions—part I. J Foot Ankle Surg 2008;47(3):180–90.
9. Wilde PH, Torode IP, Dickens DR, et al. Resection for symptomatic talocalcaneal coalition. J Bone Joint Surg Br 1994;76:797–801.
10. Giannini S, Ceccarelli F, Vannini F, et al. Operative treatment of flatfoot with talocalcaneal coalition. Clin Orthop 2003;411:178–87.
11. Mosier KM, Asher M. Tarsal coalitions and peroneal spastic flatfoot: a review. J Bone Joint Surg Am 1984;66:976–84.
12. Cowell HR, Elener V. Rigid painful flatfoot secondary to tarsal coalition. Clin Orthop 1983;177:54–60.

13. Salomão O, Napoli MM, DeCarvalho AE, et al. Talocalcaneal coalition: diagnosis and surgical management. Foot Ankle Int 1992;13:251–6.
14. Westberry DE, Davids JR, Oros W. Surgical management of symptomatic talocalcaneal coalitions by resection of the sustentaculum tali. J Pediatr Orthop 2003; 23(4):493–7.
15. Lateur LM, Van Hoe LR, Van Ghillewe KW, et al. Subtalar coalition: diagnosis with the C sign on lateral radiograph of the ankle. Radiology 1994;193:847–51.
16. Sakellariou A, Sallomi D, Janzen DL, et al. Talocalcaneal coalition: diagnosis with the C-sign on lateral radiographs of the ankle. J Bone Joint Surg Br 2000;82:574–8.
17. Kernbach KJ, Blitz NM. The presence of calcaneal fibular remodeling associated with middle facet talocalcaneal coalition: a retrospective CT review of 35 feet. Investigations involving middle facet coalitions–part II. J Foot Ankle Surg 2008; 47(4):288–94.
18. Brown RR, Rosenberg ZS, Thornhill BA. The C sign: more specific for flatfoot deformity than subtalar coalition. Skeletal Radiol 2001;30(2):84–7.
19. Leonard MA. The inheritance of tarsal coalition and its relationship to spastic flat foot. J Bone Joint Surg Br 1974;56:520–6.
20. Pfitzner W. Die Variationen im Aufbau des Fusskelets [The variations in the foot skeleton]. Morpholog Arbeit 1896;6:245–527 [in German].
21. Nalaboff KM, Schweitzer ME. MRI of tarsal coalition: frequency, distribution, and innovative signs. Bull NYU Hosp Jt Dis 2008;66(1):14–21.
22. Solomon LB, Ruhli FJ, Taylor J, et al. A dissection and computer tomograph study of tarsal coalitions in 100 cadaver feet. J Orthop Res 2003;21(2):352–8.
23. Stormont DM, Peterson HA. The relative incidence of tarsal coalition. Clin Orthop 1983;181:28–36.
24. Lahey MD, Zindrick MR, Harris EJ. A comparative study of the clinical presentation of tarsal coalitions. Clin Podiatr Med Surg 1988;5(2):341–57.
25. Harris BJ. Anomalous structures in the developing human foot [abstract]. Anat Rec 1955;121:399.
26. Wray JB, Herndon CN. Hereditary transmission of congenital coalition of the calcaneus to the navicular. J Bone Joint Surg Am 1963;45:365–72.
27. Austin FH. Symphalangism and related fusions of tarsal bones. Radiology 1951; 56:882–5.
28. Nievergelt K. Positiver Vaterschaftsnachweis auf Grunderblicher Missbildungen der Extremitaten [Inherited deformity of the extremity]. Arch Julius Klaus-Stiftung 1944;19:157–95 [in German].
29. O'Rahilly R. A survey of carpal and tarsal anomalies. J Bone Joint Surg Am 1953; 35:626–42.
30. Pearlman HS, Edkin RE, Warren RF. Familial tarsal and carpal synostosis with radial-head subluxation (Nievergelt's syndrome). J Bone Joint Surg Am 1964; 46:585–92.
31. Conway JJ, Cowell HR. Tarsal coalition: clinical significance and roentgenographic demonstration. Radiology 1969;92(4):799–811.
32. Menz HB, Gilheany MF, Landorf KB. Foot and ankle surgery in Australia: a descriptive analysis of the Medicare Benefits Schedule database, 1997–2006. J Foot Ankle Res 2008;15(1):1–10.
33. Upasani VV, Chambers RC, Mubarak SJ. Analysis of calcaneonavicular coalitions using multi-planar three dimensional computed tomography. J Child Orthop 2008;2:301–7.
34. Malicky ES, Crary JL, Houghton MJ, et al. Talocalcaneal and subfibular impingement in symptomatic flatfoot in adults. J Bone Joint Surg Am 2002;84:2005–9.

35. Cain TJ, Hyman S. Peroneal spastic flatfoot: its treatment by osteotomy of the os calcis. J Bone Joint Surg Br 1978;60(4):527–9.
36. Dwyer FC. Causes, significance and treatment of stiffness of the subtaloid joint. Proc R Soc Med 1976;69:97–102.
37. Kernbach KJ, Barkan H, Blitz NM. A critical evaluation of subtalar joint arthrosis associated with middle facet talocalcaneal coalition in 21 surgically managed patients: a retrospective CT review. Investigations involving middle facet coalitions—part III. Clin Podiatr Med Surg 2010;27(1):135–43.
38. Yen RG, Giacopelli JA, Granoff DP, et al. New nonfusion procedure for talocalcaneal coalitions with a fixed heel valgus. J Am Podiatr Med Assoc 1993;83:191–7.
39. Daumas L, Morin C, Leonard JC. Congenital tarsal synostosis. Arch Pediatr 1996; 3(9):900–5.
40. Crim J. Imaging of tarsal coalition. Radiol Clin North Am 2008;46:1017–26.
41. Swiontkowski MF, Scranton PE, Hansen S. Tarsal coalitions: long-term results of surgical treatment. J Pediatr Orthop 1983;3(3):287–92.
42. Oestreich AE, Mize WA, Crawford AH, et al. The "anteater nose": a direct sign of calcaneonavicular coalition on the lateral radiograph. J Pediatr Orthop 1987;7: 709–11.
43. Pappas AM, Miller JT. Congenital ball-and-socket ankle joints and related lower-extremity malformations. J Bone Joint Surg Am 1982;64:672–9.
44. Newman JS, Newberg AH. Congenital tarsal coalition: multimodality evaluation with emphasis on CT and MR imaging. Radiographics 2000;20:321–32.
45. Herzenberg JE, Goldner JL, Martinez S, et al. Computerized tomography of talocalcaneal tarsal coalition: a clinical and anatomic study. Foot Ankle 1986;6(6): 273–88.
46. Comfort TK, Johnson L. Resection for symptomatic talocalcaneal coalition. J Pediatr Orthop 1998;18:283–8.
47. Scranton PE. Treatment of symptomatic talocalcaneal coalition. J Bone Joint Surg Am 1987;69:533–8.
48. Varner KE, Michelson JD. Tarsal coalition in adults. Foot Ankle Int 2000;21: 669–72.
49. Taniguchi A, Tanaka Y, Kadono K, et al. C sign for diagnosis of talocalcaneal coalition. Radiology 2003;228(2):501–5.
50. Sijbrandij ES, Van Gils AP, De Lange EE, et al. Bone marrow ill-defined hyperintensities with tarsal coalition: MR imaging findings. Eur J Radiol 2002;43(1):61–5.
51. Rassi GE, Riddle EC, Kumar SJ. Arthrofibrosis involving the middle facet of the talocalcaneal joint in children and adolescents. J Bone Joint Surg Am 2005;87: 2227–31.
52. Blitz NM. Pediatric & adolescent flatfoot reconstruction in combination with middle facet talocalcaneal coalition resection. Clin Podiatr Med Surg 2010;27(1):119–33.
53. Raikin S, Cooperman DR, Thompson GH. Interposition of the split flexor hallucis longus tendon after resection of a coalition of the middle facet of the talocalcaneal joint. J Bone Joint Surg Am 1999;81(1):11–9.
54. Kumar SJ, Guille JT, Lee MS, et al. Osseous and non-osseous coalition of the middle facet of the talocalcaneal joint. J Bone Joint Surg Am 1992;74(4):529–35.
55. Kitaoka HB, Wikenheiser MA, Shaughnessy WJ, et al. Gait abnormalities following resection of the talocalcaneal coalition. J Bone Joint Surg Am 1997;79(3):369–74.
56. Olney B, Asher M. Excision of symptomatic coalition of the middle facet of the talocalcaneal joint. J Bone Joint Surg Am 1987;69(4):539–44.
57. McCormack TJ, Olney B, Asher M. Talocalcaneal coalition resection: a 10 year follow-up. J Pediatr Orthop 1997;17(1):13–5.

58. Downey MS. Tarsal coalition. In: Banks AS, Downey MS, Martin DE, et al, editors. McGlamry's comprehensive textbook of foot and ankle surgery. 3rd edition. Philadelphia: Lippincott, Williams and Wilkins; 2001. p. 993–1031.
59. Hansen ST. Progressive symptomatic flatfoot (lateral peritalar subluxation). In: Hansen ST, editor. Functional reconstruction of the foot and ankle. Philadelphia: Lippincott, Williams and Wilkins; 2000. p. 195–7.
60. Lemley F, Berlet G, Hill K, et al. Current concepts review: tarsal coalition. Foot Ankle Int 2006;27(12):1163–9.
61. Harris EJ, Vanore JV, Thomas JL, et al. Clinical practice guideline pediatric flatfoot panel. Diagnosis and treatment of pediatric flatfoot. J Foot Ankle Surg 2004;43:341–73.
62. Saltzman CL, Fehrle MJ, Cooper RR, et al. Triple arthrodesis: twenty-five and forty-four year follow up on the same patients. J Bone Joint Surg Am 1999;81: 1391–402.
63. Coester LM, Saltzman CL, Leupold J, et al. Long-term results following ankle arthrodesis for post-traumatic arthritis. J Bone Joint Surg Am 2001;83:219–28.
64. Adelaar RS, Dannelly EA, Meunier PA, et al. A long term study of triple arthrodesis in children. Orthop Clin North Am 1976;7:895–908.
65. Angus PD, Cowell HR. Triple arthrodesis. A critical long-term review. J Bone Joint Surg Br 1986;68(2):260–5.
66. Smith RW, Shen W, DeWitt S, et al. Triple arthrodesis in adults with non-paralytic disease. A minimum ten-year follow-up study. J Bone Joint Surg Am 2004;86: 2707–13.
67. Seitz DG, Carpenter EB. Triple arthrodesis in children: a ten year review. South Med J 1974;67:1420–4.

Pediatric & Adolescent Flatfoot Reconstruction in Combination with Middle Facet Talocalcaneal Coalition Resection

Neal M. Blitz, DPM, FACFAS

KEYWORDS

- Flatfoot reconstruction • Middle facet talocalcaneal coalition
- Pes planus • Tarsal coalition • Coalition-concomitant flatfoot

The concomitant rigid flatfoot that often occurs with symptomatic tarsal coalition should be considered as much as a pathologic component as the coalition itself.[1-3] Although the tarsal coalition is an "abnormal" association between two rearfoot bones, it is the effect of the restriction (partial or complete) of rearfoot motion, and position of the rearfoot (and foot), that seems to result in the cascade of pathologic symptoms.

It is undeniable that the presence of a tarsal coalition may be associated with a variety of pathologic sequelae, such as peroneal spasm; rearfoot arthrosis; equinus; traction spurring of the talonavicular and calcaneonavicular joint; ball-and-socket ankle joint; varying degrees of pes planovalgus (flatfeet); and/or abutment of the calcaneus against the fibula with pseudoarticulation (calcaneal fibular remodeling).[2,4] Although each coalition presents with a variation of these problematic sequelae (or none at all), it is unclear where the source of pain and symptoms originate, and whether or not the coalition itself is a pain producer.[1,2,5]

Traditional surgical management of tarsal coalitions by simple resection or rearfoot fusion treats complete opposite ends in the spectrum of the condition. Simple coalition resection only removes the abnormal association between the rearfoot bones in hopes that the ability to regain some degree of rearfoot motion results in resolution of symptoms but does nothing to directly treat the sequelae of coalitions (eg, the

Department of Orthopaedic Surgery, Bronx-Lebanon Hospital Center, 1650 Selwyn Avenue, Bronx, NY 10457, USA
E-mail address: nealblitz@yahoo.com

Clin Podiatr Med Surg 27 (2010) 119–133
doi:10.1016/j.cpm.2009.08.009   **podiatric.theclinics.com**

pes planus position of the foot).[1,3] In the absence of frank rearfoot arthrosis, rearfoot fusion whether isolated or as part of a triple arthrodesis treats the end result of many of the sequelae by permanently restricting rearfoot motion and realigning the foot by sacrificing vital rearfoot joints. Rearfoot fusion in a young patient population undoubtedly has long-term effects on adjacent joints. Rearfoot fusion seems to be geared toward severe malalignment. What, however, is the optimal treatment for feet in the middle of the spectrum that have a coalition with reconstructable malalignment?

Combined coalition resection and structural realignment of the foot addresses both the primary problem (the coalition) and secondary problems (aforementioned sequelae), with the latter possibly being responsible for directly producing the pain in the first place. The literature seems to be favorable for flatfoot reconstruction in association with coalition resection through (1) subtalar joint arthroereisis, (2) secondary flatfoot reconstruction, or (3) single-stage coalition resection with flatfoot reconstruction.

SIMPLE RESECTION: SOME PERSPECTIVE

Historically, surgeons focused on isolated simple coalition resection (**Fig. 1**). This is evident because the literature and studies compare outcomes between coalition resection and varying types of interpositional materials. **Table 1** identifies seven clinical studies from 1987 to 2003 reporting results of several interposition materials, such as fat, bone wax and fat, split flexor hallucis longus, no interpositional material, or bone

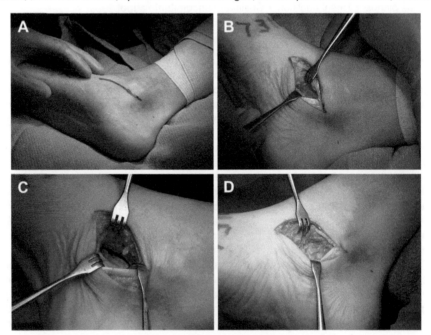

Fig. 1. Simple resection of middle facet talocalcaneal coalition with interposition of adipose tissue. (*A*) Medial curvilinear incision is placed directly over the coalition. (*B*) The coalition is defined after the posterior tibialis tendon and flexor digitorum longus tendon are reflected inferiorly. (*C*) After the coalition is resected, the posterior facet is visualized. Complete resection of the coalition restores subtalar motion and this should be seen in the operating room. (*D*) In this case, interpositional material was bone wax (not seen) and autologous adipose tissue harvested from the calf during a concomitant gastrocnemius intramuscular aponeurotic recession.

Investigator	Year	Sample size, Patients (Feet)	Age in Years at Time of Operation, Mean (Range)	Interposition Material and Concomitant Procedures	Month Follow-up, Mean (Range)	Results (Feet)
Table 1 Clinical studies of middle facet talocalcaneal coalition resection						
Olney and Asher[6]	1987	9 (10)	13.6 (10.5–22)	Fat	42 (25–91)	[b]E = 5, G = 3, F = 1, P = 1
Salomao et al[7]	1992	22 (32)	14 (10–23)	Bone wax and fat	25 (12–66)	78.1% feet completely painless; 21.8% feet achieved relief of pain; no objective pain scale used
Kumar et al[8]	1992	16 (18)	14 (7–19)	Fat, tendon, or none	48 (24–96)	[a]E = 8, G = 8, F = 1, P = 1
Kitaoka et al[9]	1997	11 (14)	17 (13–32)	Fat, tendon, or none	72 (24–156)	[a]E = 5, G = 4, F = 3, P = 2
McCormack et al[10]	1997	8 (9)	13.6 (10.5–22)	Fat	138 (120–192)	[c]E = 7, G = 0, F = 1, P = 1
Raikin et al[11]	1999	10 (14)	12 (9–16)	Split flexor hallucis longus tendon	51 (32–60)	[a]E = 11, G = 1, F = 1, P = 1
Westberry et al[12]	2003	10 (12)	12.7 (9–17.9)	Bone wax and complete sustentaculum tali excision	61.2 (18–104)	[a]E = 8, G = 3, F = 0, P = 1

Abbreviations: E, excellent; F, fair; G, good; P, poor.
[a] Denotes that the study used American Orthopaedic Foot and Ankle Society (AOFAS) ankle-hindfoot clinical rating system.
[b] Denotes that the study used the Chambers Functional Test.
[c] Denotes that the study used the Painful Foot Center questionnaire.
From Kernbach KJ, Blitz NM, Rush SM. Bilateral single-stage middle facet talocalcaneal coalition resection combined with flatfoot reconstruction: a report of 3 cases and review of the literature. Investigations involving middle facet coalitions—Part 1. J Foot Ankle Surg 2008;47:180–90; with permission.

wax with sustentaculmectomy. These studies did not evaluate specifically foot position or sequelae of coalition.[6–12]

The sample sizes of these studies range from 10 to 32 feet (average, 15 feet); involve an adolescent population; and have a mean follow-up from 25 to 138 months. Six of the aforementioned studies evaluated their postoperative results with three different scoring systems and questionnaires so it is difficult to directly compare these studies. Most of the outcomes are indeed positive with simple resection, but it becomes apparent that 8.3% to 36% of feet were overall rated as having a "fair" or "poor" result. Of the four studies that use the American Orthopaedic Foot and Ankle Society

(AOFAS) ankle-hindfoot scoring system, the percentages of "fair and/or poor" outcomes are 8.3%, 11%, 22%, and 36% of feet.[8,9,11,12] Because these studies evaluated some degree of the patients' perspective with regard to pain, this suggests that the coalition itself may not be the primary source of pain, and furthermore suggests that there is more to tarsal coalition surgery than the pure resection of the coalition. Although interposition material is indeed important to prevent regrowth of the coalition, it is only part of the pathologic problems associated with coalition.

REARFOOT ARTHRODESIS

Rearfoot arthrodesis has been advocated for the treatment of tarsal coalition when rearfoot arthrosis is present and when severe pes planovalgus deformity exists.[4,13] Although rearfoot arthrodesis truly solves the coalition and the malalignment issues, the procedure is not without its downside and long-term degenerating effects on adjacent joints.[14,15] Studies have not emerged that specifically look at outcomes after rearfoot fusion with coalition resection in the absence of arthritis. This is likely because the guidelines that direct a surgeon to rearfoot fusion are blurred, and it is not entirely clear when rearfoot fusion is most appropriate. As such, in the absence of arthrosis, rearfoot fusion has been directed toward the "very" flat foot.

In 2004, a clinical practice guideline on diagnosis and treatment of pediatric flatfoot was developed by the Clinical Practice Guideline Pediatric Flatfoot Panel of the American College of Foot and Ankle Surgeons, based on the "consensus of current clinic practice and review of the clinical literature," stating the following: "resection of the coalition may be indicated for individuals without significant deformity or arthrosis. In some cases, arthrodesis may be the procedure of choice."[13] Additionally, "in children with foot deformity, osteotomy should be performed in conjunction with resection. If significant arthritic changes are found, arthrodesis should be considered. Isolated talocalcaneal arthrodesis is indicated for subtalar coalitions. If peritalar degeneration is evident, triple arthrodesis may also be indicated." Although the clinical practice guideline clearly identifies the surgical treatment possibilities, specific guidelines for surgical treatment of the foot deformity seem to have been beyond the focus of the practice guideline. This generality does allow for some surgical flexibility for surgeons managing this "under" understood entity.

Overall, it seems from the literature and practice habits that surgeons identify factors that favor or sway one into performing or not performing a rearfoot fusion. Some investigators have looked at middle facet coalition size as a function of total subtalar joint involvement. Scranton[16] has suggested that when greater than 50% of the subtalar joint is involved then arthrodesis be performed. Luhmann and Schoenecker[5] demonstrated that a statistically significant poorer outcome was associated with a talocalcaneal coalition involving greater than 50% of posterior facet surface (identified on CT), although they did point out that "talocalcaneal coalition size does not absolutely predict post-resection outcome." Comfort and Johnson[17] achieved a 77% excellent or good outcome after resection of 17 coalitions that involved less than one third of the entire subtalar joint surface, measured on CT. Kumar and colleagues[8] advocate coalition resection regardless of the extent of the middle facet involvement. In a previous publication I have recommended that, in the absence of talonavicular joint arthritis, isolated realignment subtalar joint arthrodesis should be performed when CT demonstrates greater than 50% involvement of the posterior facet and significant subtalar arthrosis (spurring and subtalar cysts).[1] Interestingly, there does not seem to be a distinction between type of coalition (osseous or fibrous) that directs a surgeon toward fusion or resection. Nonetheless, it does seem that coalition size may play a role in the decision process as to whether or not fusion should be performed, however, size should be taken into account with the other sequelae of coalitions.

UNDERSTANDING COALITION-ASSOCIATED REARFOOT ARTHROSIS

Rearfoot arthrosis in conjunction with middle facet coalition has been an indication for isolated, double, or triple arthrodesis. The posterior facet of the subtalar joint is the most common joint to be affected by arthritic degeneration, whereas the talonavicular joint often develops nonarthritic traction spurring. Intraoperatively, surgeons may evaluate the articular cartilage of the posterior facet for arthritic changes, but this does not help with preoperative decision-making (**Fig. 2**). Preoperatively, surgeons use CT scans to better determine the extent of the arthrosis (besides coalition size) and look for joint space narrowing and cystic changes.[1,7,12,18] Although the definition of rearfoot arthrosis in the context of middle facet coalition has been somewhat vague or loosely observer dependent, the mere presence of arthritis often dictates whether or not fusion should be performed.[13]

Until recently, the ability to stage the degree or severity of concomitant posterior facet arthrosis on CT did not exist.[19] Included within this edition of the Clinics is a newly developed CT staging system to better categorize and define the extent of coalition-associated subtalar arthrosis (**Fig. 3**). This classification system was developed as part of a retrospective research study that specifically looked at 12 years of data in 12 surgeon's logs, identifying 21 patients (35 feet) with symptomatic middle facet coalitions who had at least one foot surgery for coalition management, and a preoperative CT available for review. Studies that evaluate intraobserver and interobserver differences with this newly developed staging system do not exist. Additionally, the staging of arthrosis was based purely on radiographic criteria; however, scans evaluated were patients with coalition-associated symptoms.

Posterior facet arthrosis was graded into three stages and the following distribution of arthrosis was indentified: stage I (normal-mild), 57.1%; stage II (moderate), 34.3%; stage III (severe), 8.6%. The mean age of patients with stage I, II, and III arthrosis was 14, 25, and 41 years, respectively. The association of stage and age was statistically significant ($P = .001$). Nearly 60% of feet had normal-mild degenerative changes and when combined with moderate degenerative changes accounts for 91.4%, and in patients younger than a mean age of 25. Severe end-stage arthrosis was the least common and occurred in older patients (mean age, 41 years).

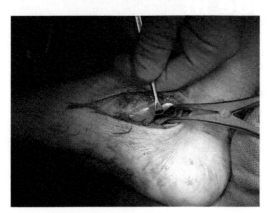

Fig. 2. Once the coalition is resected, the posterior facet may be visualized and inspected for signs of arthrosis. A lamina spreader is useful in spreading this joint open.

Blitz & Kernbach CT Staging System of Posterior Facet Arthrosis Associated with Middle Facet Talocalcaneal Coalition

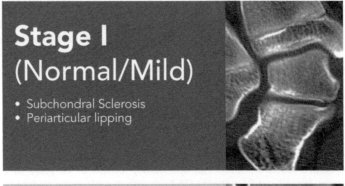

Stage I (Normal/Mild)

- Subchondral Sclerosis
- Periarticular lipping

Stage II (Moderate)

- Articular erosions
- Subchondral cysts
- Asymmetric joint narrowing
- Osteophyte formation

Stage III (Severe)

- Complete loss/obliteration of joint space
- Destruction accounts for > 50% posterior facet surface
- Exuberant osteophytes
- Significant sclerosis

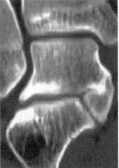

Fig. 3. Newly developed Blitz and Kernbach CT staging system is a guide for surgeons to grade the extent of coalition-associated posterior facet arthrosis.

Whether or not this CT classification translates into clinical practice to clarify indications for simple resection, resection with flatfoot reconstruction, or fusion remains to be seen. This CT study allows for surgeons to better understand the range of arthritic changes that may occur within the posterior facet and now classify and categorize the extent. Moreover the results of that CT study identified, in the sample size of 35 feet, that end-stage radiographic arthrosis occurs in less than 10% of coalition-associated subtalar arthrosis and implies that fusion is completely appropriate in these arthritic feet. Is fusion the answer in the other 90% where arthrosis is less severe? In the case of the 60% or so of normal or mild degeneration, fusion on the basis of arthritic changes seems to be less appropriate. The difficultly lies in the 34% where there are moderate arthritic changes, and the surgeon has to determine fusion over resection or flatfoot reconstruction. It is in these cases that the position of the foot and sequelae of clinical presentation are most important.

THE COALITION CONCOMITANT FLATFOOT: A PATHOLOGIC ENTITY

Symptomatic flatfoot in the absence of tarsal coalition is considered a pathologic entity worthy of surgical realignment, yet in the presence of tarsal coalition the flatfoot has been largely ignored, and often an afterthought. Correction of the coalition-concomitant associated pes planus is classically considered as a secondary procedure as part of a revision surgery once isolated resection of a tarsal coalition has progressed to failure.[5,12] Westberry and colleagues[12] performed complete excision of the sustentaculum tali in 12 coalitions (10 patients), and identified that residual pes planovalgus deformity was the source of pain in one patient, who subsequently underwent flatfoot reconstruction with a lateral column lengthening after the index resection. Two recent studies have also emerged suggesting poorer outcomes associated with isolated resection in the presence of severe heel valgus (>16 degrees and >21 degrees, respectively).[4,18] Collins[20] acknowledged that foot pain may exist after isolated coalition resection if orthotics are not worn postoperatively.

In regard to middle facet tarsal coalition, the lateral position of the heel on the leg (rearfoot valgus) can result in pathologic and morphologic changes of the calcaneus, fibula, and subtalar joint. Perhaps this malalignment is responsible for the arthritic degeneration of the subtalar joint, rather than the mere presence of the coalition itself. Recently, in a previous publication, I studied and reported on the abutment of the calcaneus and fibula as potential source of symptoms, a condition that has not been previously described, and termed the condition "calcaneal fibular remodeling," which characterizes the morphologic pseudoarticulation that seems to occur between the calcaneus and fibula, in some cases, as a result of the fixed heel valgus (**Fig. 4**).[2] Depending on the severity of the hindfoot valgus, spurring and cystic changes may occur. These objective radiographic findings further illustrate that valgus position of the heel may result in a pathologic degenerative process. It is unclear if calcaneal fibular remodeling actually represents a painful condition on its own and further investigations into this area are welcome.

COALITION RESECTION WITH FLATFOOT RECONSTRUCTION

Coalition resection with flatfoot reconstruction is not an entirely new concept, and few published reports are available. Yen and colleagues[21] performed an opening wedge calcaneal osteotomy of the tuber to correct rigid calcaneal valgus associated with a middle facet coalition in a single case. Cain and Hyman[22] described an isolated medial closing wedge of the calcaneus of 14 peroneal spastic flatfeet (some with tarsal coalition). In the series by Westberry and coworkers[12] of sustentaculumectomy in

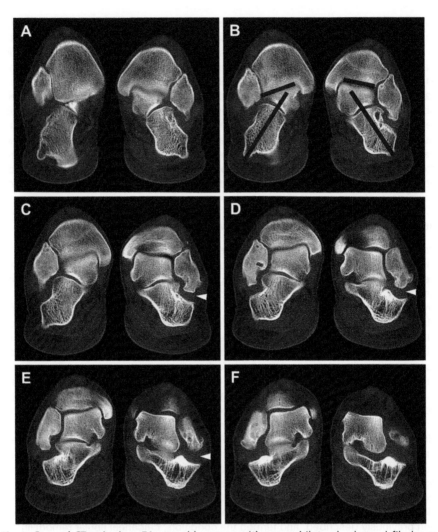

Fig. 4. Coronal CT series in a 51-year old woman with severe bilateral calcaneal fibular remodeling associated with middle facet tarsal coalition. (*A–F*) Cross-sections go from most proximal (*A*) to distal (*F*). (*B*) The fixed valgus position of the hindfoot is responsible for the morphologic changes. The *blue lines* bisecting the heel and tibia demonstrate the heel valgus. (*C, D*) *Red arrowheads* illustrate the abutment that may occur. (*D*) Note the "cup-like" changes and pseudoarticulation.

12 coalitions (10 patients), four patients had concomitant procedures to correct foot alignment: one patient underwent a Dwyer closing wedge calcaneal osteotomy, another a gastrocnemius-soleus recession, and yet another patient had bilateral calcaneocuboid distraction arthrodeses. Separately, Downey[23] Lepow and Richman[24] have combined arthroereisis with middle facet coalition resection to improve foot alignment in separate case reports. Giannini and colleagues[3] combined single-stage tarsal coalition resection and subtalar arthroereisis using a bioresorbable implant in 14 feet in young patients (median age, 14 years old). The patients with the worst results were older, and the investigators suggested that arthroereisis be performed before the

age of 14 to allow for bone remodeling. They also advocated that hindfoot realignment with subtalar joint arthrodesis was preferred (over subtalar arthroereisis) in the skeletally mature patient.

Recently, in a previous publication, I studied and reported on bilateral single-stage middle facet talocalcaneal coalition resection combined with flatfoot reconstruction in three cases (six feet).[1] The retrospective review of six feet demonstrated excellent clinical results because the mean postoperative AOFAS ankle-hindfoot score was 94.33 ± 2.81 points. These feet also demonstrated statistically improved median radiographic angles for calcaneal inclination, Meary's, and anteroposterior talar–first metatarsal angles. Moreover, the patients in this review had bilateral reconstruction where one foot was corrected followed by at least 6 months before the contralateral correction. From the patients' perspective, if they had not been pleased with the functional result of their first surgery then they would likely not have undergone contralateral correction. This small retrospective study suggests that there is a role for single-stage concomitant flatfoot reconstruction combined with middle facet talocalcaneal coalition resection.

Figs. 5–10 illustrate several patients who have undergone a single-stage middle facet talocalcaneal coalition resection combined with flatfoot reconstruction. From a pure radiographic standpoint these feet demonstrate improved structure, some cases more dramatic than others. It may be difficult or impossible to achieve a perfect radiographic alignment in all cases, especially when severe pes planus exists, and surgeons try not to perform rearfoot fusions. The goal is to improve the overall alignment by avoiding rearfoot fusion in this young patient population, especially when presented with skeletally immature patients.

SURGICAL TREATMENT GUIDELINES

Guidelines and a treatment algorithm that specifically consider the pes planus as a pathologic component of tarsal coalition when considering reconstruction have

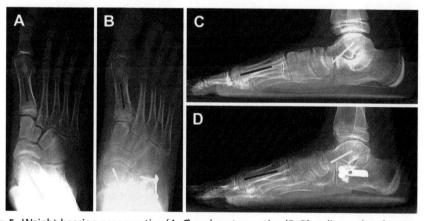

Fig. 5. Weight-bearing preoperative (*A, C*) and postoperative (*B, D*) radiographs of a 12-year and 4-month old boy who underwent right middle facet talocalcaneal coalition resection and flatfoot reconstruction (tendo-Achilles lengthening and Evans calcaneal osteotomy). The postoperative AOFAS score was 92. Improved talo–first metatarsal angle (*yellow and blue lines*) and calcaneal inclination angle (*red triangle*) are evident. (*From* Kernbach KJ, Blitz NM, Rush SM. Bilateral single-stage middle facet talocalcaneal coalition resection combined with flatfoot reconstruction: a report of 3 cases and review of the literature. Investigations involving middle facet coalitions—Part 1. J Foot Ankle Surg 2008;47:180–90; with permission.)

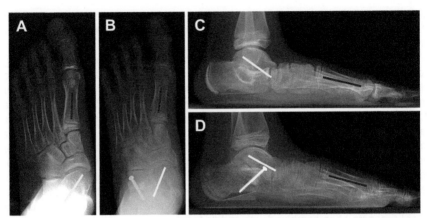

Fig. 6. Weight-bearing preoperative (*A, C*) and postoperative (*B, D*) radiographs of a 12-year and 10-month old boy who underwent left middle facet talocalcaneal coalition resection and flatfoot reconstruction (tendo-Achilles lengthening and Evans calcaneal osteotomy). The postoperative AOFAS score was 90. Improved talo–first metatarsal angle (*yellow and blue lines*) and calcaneal inclination angle (*red triangle*) are evident. (*From* Kernbach KJ, Blitz NM, Rush SM. Bilateral single-stage middle facet talocalcaneal coalition resection combined with flatfoot reconstruction: a report of 3 cases and review of the literature. Investigations involving middle facet coalitions—Part 1. J Foot Ankle Surg 2008;47:180–90; with permission.)

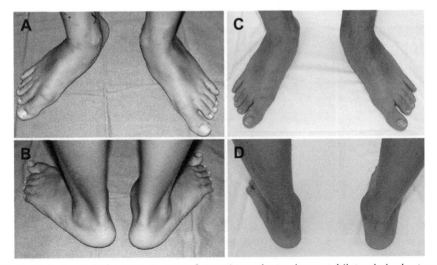

Fig. 7. Clinical weight-bearing images of a patient who underwent bilateral single-stage middle facet talocalcaneal coalition resection with flatfoot reconstruction. These clinical images correspond to radiographs in **Figs. 5 and 6**. Preoperative (*A, C*) and postoperative (*B, D*). (*From* Kernbach KJ, Blitz NM, Rush SM. Bilateral single-stage middle facet talocalcaneal coalition resection combined with flatfoot reconstruction: a report of 3 cases and review of the literature. Investigations involving middle facet coalitions—Part 1. J Foot Ankle Surg 2008;47:180–90; with permission.)

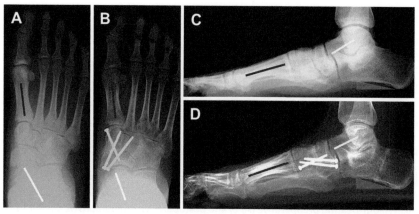

Fig. 8. Weight-bearing preoperative (*A, C*) and postoperative (*B, D*) radiographs of a 16-year and 8-month old girl who underwent right middle facet talocalcaneal coalition resection and flatfoot reconstruction (tendo-Achilles lengthening, medializing calcaneal osteotomy, Evans calcaneal osteotomy, naviculocuneiform arthrodesis, and posterior tibial tendon augmentation with flexor digitorum longus). The postoperative AOFAS score was 97. Improved talo–first metatarsal angle (*yellow and blue lines*) and calcaneal inclination angle (*red triangle*) are evident. (*From* Kernbach KJ, Blitz NM, Rush SM. Bilateral single-stage middle facet talocalcaneal coalition resection combined with flatfoot reconstruction: a report of 3 cases and review of the literature. Investigations involving middle facet coalitions—Part 1. J Foot Ankle Surg 2008;47:180–90; with permission.)

been recently suggested (**Table 2**).[1] Coalitions are categorized in three types depending on the presence of pes planus or hindfoot arthrosis. Type I coalitions are not associated with pes planus or rearfoot arthrosis. Type II coalitions occur with pes planus but without hindfoot arthrosis. Type III coalitions occur with pes planus and hindfoot arthrosis. Depending on the presence of pes planus and rearfoot arthrosis, surgical

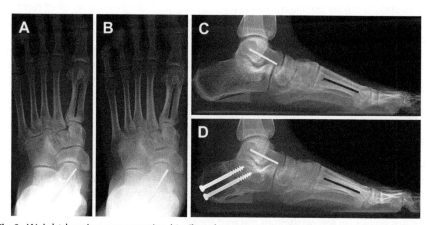

Fig. 9. Weight-bearing preoperative (*A, C*) and postoperative (*B, D*) radiographs of a 17-year and 8-month old girl who underwent left middle facet talocalcaneal coalition resection and flatfoot reconstruction (tendo-Achilles lengthening, medializing calcaneal osteotomy). The postoperative AOFAS score was 97. Improved talo–first metatarsal angle (*yellow and blue lines*) and calcaneal inclination angle (*red triangle*) are evident.

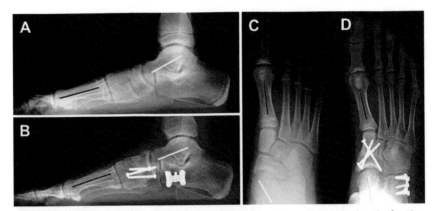

Fig. 10. Weight-bearing preoperative (*A, C*) and postoperative radiographs (*B, D*) of a 13-year and 5-month old boy who underwent right middle facet talocalcaneal coalition resection and flatfoot reconstruction (gastrocnemius intramuscular aponeurotic lengthening, naviculocuneiform arthrodesis, and Evans calcaneal osteotomy). The postoperative AOFAS score was 95. Improved talo–first metatarsal angle (*yellow and blue lines*) and calcaneal inclination angle (*red triangle*) are evident (*From* Kernbach KJ, Blitz NM, Rush SM. Bilateral single-stage middle facet talocalcaneal coalition resection combined with flatfoot reconstruction: a report of 3 cases and review of the literature. Investigations involving middle facet coalitions—Part 1. J Foot Ankle Surg 2008;47:180–90; with permission.)

recommendations are made. This guideline is merely a framework to assist surgeons in the decision-making process when considering flat foot reconstruction or rearfoot fusions in combination with coalition resection.

SURGICAL MANAGEMENT OF TYPE I

In type I, simple resection of the coalition is the treatment of choice. Because no structural foot deformity exists and there is no associated rearfoot arthrosis, rearfoot fusions should not be considered. Notwithstanding that, surgeons may elect rearfoot fusion purely based on the size of coalition. In this subset of patients, equinus may coexist and tendo-Achilles lengthening or gastrocnemius recession (gastrocnemius intramuscular aponeurotic recession) may be concomitantly performed.[1,25] In my experience, more severe coalition-associated pes planus is associated with a more advanced equinus contracture that involves both gastrocnemius and soleus, and tendo-Achilles lengthening is indicated. These decisions are based on the clinical presentation and surgeon experience.

SURGICAL MANAGEMENT OF TYPE II

The type II coalition is the most difficult of the coalitions to assess and formulate a treatment plan. Type II presents with varying degrees of pes planus (from mild to severe) and without rearfoot arthrosis. The decision-making process to decide rearfoot fusion in this group should not be made on the presence of arthrosis; rather, decisions are based on the position of the foot (or coalition size).

The method of flatfoot reconstruction should be based on the same principles of flatfoot reconstruction for those patients without concomitant coalition, and based on the plane of deformity, skeletal maturity, and clinical examination.[1,26] Mild and moderate pes planus may respond to arthroereisis. Fusion of nonessential midfoot

Table 2
Blitz and Kernbach proposed classification and surgical treatment algorithms for symptomatic middle facet talocalcaneal coalitions (TCC)

Type of Coalition	Associated Pathology	Intervention
I	TCC + no pes planus without rearfoot arthrosis	Resection of the coalition
II	TCC + mild pes planus without rearfoot arthrosis	Resection ± flatfoot[a] reconstruction
	TCC + moderate pes planus without rearfoot arthrosis	Resection ± flatfoot[a] reconstruction
	TCC + severe pes planus without rearfoot arthrosis	Resection ± flatfoot[a] reconstruction or appropriate rearfoot arthrodesis
III	TCC + pes planus with symptomatic subtalar arthrosis	Subtalar fusion ± flatfoot[a] reconstruction or triple arthrodesis
	TCC + pes planus with symptomatic subtalar and talonavicular arthrosis	Subtalar and talonavicular fusion ± flatfoot[a] reconstruction or triple arthrodesis
	TCC + pes planus with symptomatic subtalar, talonavicular, and calcaneocuboid arthrosis	Triple arthrodesis

Abbreviation: TCC, talocalcaneal coalitions.

[a] Flatfoot reconstruction may involve one or a combination of the following depending on the plane of deformity and skeletal maturity: subtalar arthroereisis, medializing calcaneal osteotomy, Evans osteotomy or distraction calcaneocuboid arthrodesis, gastrocnemius recession, tendo-Achilles lengthening, or medial column procedure or fusion.

From Kernbach KJ, Blitz NM, Rush SM. Bilateral single-stage middle facet talocalcaneal coalition resection combined with flatfoot reconstruction: a report of 3 cases and review of the literature. Investigations involving middle facet coalitions—Part 1. J Foot Ankle Surg 2008;47:180–90; with permission

joints may be indicated if radiographic evidence of arch collapse is evident at these locations. A medializing calcaneal osteotomy may be used with frontal plane heel valgus, which is often visualized on the CT scan. With regard to forefoot abduction, surgeons may need to consider between an Evans calcaneal osteotomy and a calcaneocuboid distraction arthrodesis. In a small series of six feet treated with coalition resection and flatfoot reconstruction, four of the six patients underwent Evans calcaneal osteotomy.[1] In a skeletally immature patient with a severe pes planus, the correction may have been radiographically better with calcaneocuboid distraction fusions, but we elected to attempt a joint-sparing method with the Evans osteotomy. Clinically, the overall alignment of the foot was not perfect but was significantly improved from the preoperative state and correction afforded pain resolution. The precise method of flatfoot reconstruction may be surgeon dependent and, perhaps with improved anatomic alignment in a growing patient, function may be improved over the course of musculoskeletal development and maturity.[1]

Because the definition of arthrosis is vague it should be understood that, within the type II group, mild or moderate posterior facet arthrosis (stage I or II, respectively) may exist and surgeons may have to consider just how much of a contribution the stage II arthrosis actually makes to the pain cascade as one considers flatfoot reconstruction. Studies do not exist that grade the stage of posterior facet arthrosis and outcomes for any intervention whatsoever, because the concept of staging-grading the posterior facet arthrosis with coalition is new.[19] It should be pointed out, however, that most feet (91.4%) in the aforementioned study had normal-mild degenerative changes or moderate degenerative changes indicating that some degree of posterior facet degeneration seems to coexist with coalitions, so the challenge that surgeons face is to decipher if the moderate degenerative changes are "fusion" worthy. If mild to moderate pes planovalgus is present, and moderate arthritic changes exist, then flatfoot reconstruction should be strongly considered in young patients. Severe pes planus with moderate arthrosis may be theoretically more amenable to fusion, but it was demonstrated that on a small scale simply improving the overall foot alignment improves the postoperative outcome, as measured on AOFAS scores.[1] This is an area of future investigation.

SURGICAL MANAGEMENT OF TYPE III

In type III, the presence of frank arthrosis clearly supersedes any malalignment issues, and the indications for fusion are very clear. The clinical and radiographic studies determine the need for isolated, double, or triple arthrodesis. Isolated subtalar fusion may be performed in conjunction with flatfoot reconstruction when the talonavicular or calcaneocuboid joints are pristine or minimally degenerative.

SUMMARY

There seems to be a resurgence of interest in the surgical management of middle facet coalitions, especially as it relates to concomitant pes planovalgus. As further studies emerge illustrating that the concomitant flatfoot is indeed a pathologic entity, the concept of concomitant correction may become more mainstream. It should be remembered that surgically addressing the concomitant pes planovalgus is not an entirely new concept. Recent studies support the concomitant single-stage treatment of the flatfoot with arthroereisis or flatfoot reconstruction. Guidelines presented within this article may aid the surgeon when attempting to surgically manage the coalition-associated flatfoot.

REFERENCES

1. Kernbach KJ, Blitz NM, Rush SM. Bilateral single-stage middle facet talocalcaneal coalition resection combined with flatfoot reconstruction: a report of 3 cases and review of the literature. Investigations involving middle facet coalitions—part 1. J Foot Ankle Surg 2008;47(3):180–90.
2. Kernbach KJ, Blitz NM. The presence of calcaneal fibular remodeling associated with middle facet talocalcaneal coalition: a retrospective CT review of 35 feet. Investigations involving middle facet coalitions – part II. J Foot Ankle Surg 2008;47(4):321–5.
3. Giannini S, Ceccarelli F, Vannini F, et al. Operative treatment of flatfoot with talocalcaneal coalition. Clin Orthop 2003;411:178–87.
4. Downey MS. Tarsal coalition. In: Banks AS, Downey MS, Martin DE, et al, editors. McGlamry's comprehensive textbook of foot and ankle surgery. 3rd edition. Philadelphia: Lippincott Williams and Wilkins; 2001. p. 993–1031.
5. Luhmann SJ, Schoenecker PL. Symptomatic talocalcaneal coalition resection: indications and results. J Pediatr Orthop 1998;186:748–54.
6. Olney B, Asher M. Excision of symptomatic coalition of the middle facet of the talocalcaneal joint. J Bone Joint Surg Am 1987;69(4):539–44.
7. Salomao O, Napoli MM, DeCarvalho AE, et al. Talocalcaneal coalition: diagnosis and surgical management. Foot Ankle Int 1992;13:251–6.

8. Kumar SJ, Guille JT, Lee MS, et al. Osseous and non-osseous coalition of the middle facet of the talocalcaneal joint. J Bone Joint Surg Am 1992;74(4):529–35.

9. Kitaoka HB, Wikenheiser MA, Shaughnessy WJ, et al. Gait abnormalities following resection of the talocalcaneal coalition. J Bone Joint Surg Am 1997;79(3):369–74.

10. McCormack TJ, Olney B, Asher M. Talocalcaneal coalition resection: a 10 year follow-up. J Pediatr Orthop 1997;171:13–5.

11. Raikin S, Cooperman DR, Thompson GH. Interposition of the Split flexor hallucis longus tendon after resection of a coalition of the middle facet of the talocalcaneal joint. J Bone Joint Surg Am 1999;81(1):11–9.

12. Westberry DE, Davids JR, Oros W. Surgical management of symptomatic talocalcaneal coalitions by resection of the sustentaculum tali. J Pediatr Orthop 2003; 234:493–7.

13. Harris EJ, Vanore JV, Thomas JL. Diagnosis and treatment of pediatric flatfoot. J Foot Ankle Surg 2004;43(6):341–73.

14. Saltzman CL, Fehrle MJ, Cooper RR, et al. Triple arthrodesis: twenty-five and forty-four year follow up on the same patients. J Bone Joint Surg Am 1999;81: 1391–402.

15. Coester LM, Saltzman CL, Leupold J, et al. Long-term results following ankle arthrodesis for post-traumatic arthritis. J Bone Joint Surg Am 2001;83:219–28.

16. Scranton PE. Treatment of symptomatic talocalcaneal coalition. J Bone Joint Surg Am 1987;69:533–8.

17. Comfort TK, Johnson L. Resection for symptomatic talocalcaneal coalition. J Pediatr Orthop 1998;18:283–8.

18. Wilde PH, Torode IP, Dickens DR, et al. Resection for symptomatic talocalcaneal coalition. J Bone Joint Surg Br 1994;76:797–801.

19. Kernbach KJ, Blitz NM. A critical evaluation of subtalar joint arthrosis associated with middle facet talocalcaneal coalition in 21 surgically managed patients: a retrospective ct review. investigations involving middle facet coalitions – part III. Clin Podiatr Med Surg 2010;27:135–43.

20. Collins B. Tarsal coalitions: a new surgical procedure. Clin Podiatr Med Surg 1987;41:75–98.

21. Yen RG, Giacopelli JA, Granoff DP, et al. New nonfusion procedure for talocalcaneal coalitions with a fixed heel valgus. J Am Podiatr Med Assoc 1993;83:191–7.

22. Cain TJ, Hyman S. Peroneal spastic flatfoot: its treatment by osteotomy of the os calcis. J Bone Joint Surg Br 1978;60(4):527–9.

23. Downey MS. Resection of middle facet talocalcaneal coalitions. In: Miller SJ, Mahan KT, Yu GV, et al, editors. Reconstructive Surgery of the foot and leg: update '98. Tucker (GA): Podiatry Institute; 1998. p. 1–5.

24. Lepow GM, Richman HM. Talocalcaneal coalition: a unique treatment approach in case report. Podiatr Tracts 1988;1:38–43.

25. Blitz NM, Rush SM. The gastrocnemius intramuscular aponeurotic recession: a simplified method of gastrocnemius recession. J Foot Ankle Surg 2007;462: 133–8.

26. Mosca VS. Calcaneal lengthening for valgus deformity of the hindfoot: results in children who had severe, symptomatic flatfoot and skewfoot. J Bone Joint Surg Am 1995;774:500–12.

A Critical Evaluation of Subtalar Joint Arthrosis Associated with Middle Facet Talocalcaneal Coalition in 21 Surgically Managed Patients: A Retrospective Computed Tomography Review. Investigations Involving Middle Facet Coalitions—Part III

Klaus J. Kernbach, DPM[a], Howard Barkan, DrPH[b],
Neal M. Blitz, DPM, FACFAS[c],*

KEYWORDS

- Tarsal coalition • Subtalar joint arthrosis • Pes planus
- Middle facet talocalcaneal coalition
- Coalition concomitant arthritis

Identifying subtalar joint arthrosis (posterior facet) is of utmost importance when patients with symptomatic middle facet talocalcaneal coalition (TCC) are managed surgically.[1–5] Subtalar arthritis often dictates whether a rearfoot fusion should be

Financial disclosures, None reported; Conflicts of interest, None reported.
[a] Department of Podiatry, Kaiser Foundation Hospital, 975 Sereno Drive, Vallejo, CA 94589, USA
[b] Joint Medical Program, School of Public Health, University of Califoria, Berkeley, Berkeley, CA 94720, USA
[c] Department of Orthopaedic Surgery, Bronx-Lebanon Hospital Center, 1650 Selwyn Avenue, Bronx, NY 10457, USA
* Corresponding author.
E-mail address: nealblitz@yahoo.com (N.M. Blitz).

performed or not.[2] However, its absence allows for the simple resection of the coalition.[2,6,7] If pes planovalgus is present, the resection may be combined with single-stage flatfoot correction.[1,2,8,9] Computerized axial tomography (CT) is necessary to evaluate the type of coalition (osseous vs fibrous), extent of the coalition, and the presence of subtalar joint arthrosis.[2,9,10] However, no specific guidelines exist to stage the degree or severity of any concomitant subtalar arthrosis. This investigation presents a CT staging system (**Table 1**) for subtalar arthrosis, and examines the association of this staged severity with the type of middle facet TCC.

Better understanding of the extent of subtalar joint arthrosis associated with middle facet coalition will help guide the surgeon in recommending a coalition resection or subtalar joint fusion.[2,9] In a patient with symptomatic middle facet TCC and nonarthritic posterior facet, a subtalar joint salvage procedure, such as isolated resection of the coalition with or without additional procedures, is indicated to improve any segmental alignment of the foot.[1,2,9,10] However, a subtalar joint salvage procedure is not indicated in a patient with symptomatic middle facet TCC and an arthritic or nearly ankylosed posterior facet.[1,2] A subtalar joint arthrodesis with appropriate correction of any additional segmental misalignment may be more appropriate.[2,9] Avoiding rearfoot fusion of essential joints in young patients with middle facet TCC is important, as the consequences of rearfoot fusion may include painful subsequent arthritis of the adjacent joints.[11,12] In this investigation, the extent of preoperative subtalar joint (posterior facet) arthrosis has been objectively evaluated by an original predefined grading system in a large cohort of patients with middle facet TCC who were managed surgically for at least 1 foot.

MATERIALS AND METHODS

The authors conducted a retrospective review of 12 years' data in 12 surgeons' logs of patients who had middle facet TCC identified on preoperative CT and were treated by surgical management. Surgical management of the TCC was defined as operative intervention that may have included 1 of the following procedures: simple resection of the coalition, rearfoot arthrodesis, or combined single-stage flatfoot reconstruction with middle facet coalition resection. The authors identified 21 patients with preoperative CT scans of middle facet TCC who had at least 1 foot surgery for coalition management. If a patient was found to have bilateral middle facet TCC on CT and if only 1 foot was operated on, then the contralateral nonsurgically treated foot was also included in this review. Patients who did not have even 1 surgery for middle facet

Table 1	
Blitz and Kernbach CT staging system of the posterior facet arthrosis associated with middle facet TCC	
Stage	**CT Finding**
Stage I (normal/mild)	• Subchondral sclerosis • Periarticular lipping • Minimal or no joint space narrowing
Stage II (moderate)	• Joint narrowing • Osteophyte formation • Subchondral cysts • Articular erosions
Stage III (severe/end-stage)	• Complete loss/obliteration of joint space • Destruction >50% posterior facet surface • Exuberant osteophytes • Significant sclerosis

TCC were excluded from the study. Patients for whom magnetic resonance imaging (MRI) was completed without CT scan were also excluded from this study, as the authors deemed MRI to be inconclusive in some cases for scrutinizing the extent of coalition and arthrosis.

For each patient, CT scans were reviewed electronically by the authors (KJK and NMB). All CT scans used a slice width between 1 and 4.5 mm, with a mean of 2.4 mm. The CT scans were evaluated for the type of middle facet TCC (osseous vs fibrous) and the presence of middle facet TCC on the contralateral foot if scans were available. Coalitions were defined by significant middle facet joint irregularity (consistent with a fibrous coalition) or trabecular bridging at the middle facet (consistent with an osseous coalition) from the talus to the calcaneus.

Subtalar (posterior facet talocalcaneal) joint arthrosis was reviewed and graded in each foot with the newly developed classification (see **Table 1**). In this new classification, Stage I (normal/mild) posterior facet arthrosis was defined by subchondral sclerosis, periarticular lipping, and minimal or no joint space narrowing (**Fig. 1**). Stage II (moderate) posterior facet arthrosis was defined by joint narrowing, osteophyte formation, subchondral cysts, and articular erosions (**Fig. 2**). Stage III (severe or "end-stage") posterior facet arthrosis was defined by complete loss or obliteration of joint space, destruction accounting for more than 50% of the posterior facet surface, exuberant osteophytes, and significant sclerosis (**Fig. 3**). The same CT scans used for coalition evaluation were used to identify the posterior facet arthrosis. In all instances, the arthrosis was most easily identified on the coronal CT slices. Sagittal and transverse slices were also evaluated in all cases for further elucidation.

Standard descriptive statistics were used to characterize the patient population. Correlation and regression statistics were used to explore the association between scalar demographic measures and stage. Standard bivariate inferential statistics were used to examine the association of coalition type with predictor variables. Finally, multinomial logistic regression was used to explore and model the association between coalition type and stage.[13] All analyses were conducted using SPSS Statistics 17.0 (Release 17.0.0; June 17, 2008).

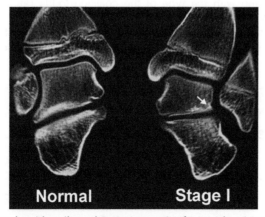

Fig. 1. 13-year-old male with unilateral Stage I posterior facet arthrosis and fibrous coalition (not completely depicted in this slice). The contralateral side does not have a coalition, and the subtalar joint is normal. Note the subtle periarticular lipping (*arrow*) and the slightest differences in joint space between the 2 feet.

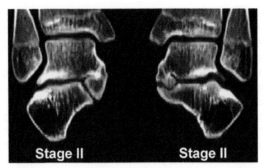

Fig. 2. 13-year-old female with bilateral Stage II posterior facet arthrosis and fibrous coalitions. Note the presence of posterior facet articular erosions (*asterisks*) and joint space narrowing.

RESULTS

The results are tabulated in **Table 2**. A total of 35 feet in 21 patients fulfilled the inclusion criteria. Eleven patients (52.4%; 95% confidence interval [CI], 29.8%–74.3%) were male and 10 (47.6%; 95% CI, 25.7%–70.2%) were female. The average age of the feet at the time of CT was 20.2 years (95% CI, 15.0–25.3 years). The average age of the male patients was 17.7 years (95% CI, 11.6–23.8 years), and the average age of the female patients was 22.5 years (95% CI, 13.9–31.1 years). The difference in average age between the male and female patients was not statistically significant (P = .35, not significant). There were 21 left feet (60%; 95% CI, 42.1%–76.1%) and 14 right feet (40%; 95% CI, 23.9%–57.9%).

Stage I arthrosis was identified in 20 feet (57.1%; 95% CI, 39.4%–73.7%), Stage II arthrosis in 12 feet (34.3%; 95% CI, 19.1%–52.2%), and Stage III arthrosis in 3 feet (8.6%; 95% CI, 1.8%–23.1%). The mean age of patients with Stage I, II, and III arthrosis was 14, 25, and 41 years, respectively. Patient's age at the time of CT scan is positively associated with the stage of posterior facet arthrosis (regression slope, 0.547; Student's t, 3.750; P = .001). All of the feet with Stage III arthrosis had fibrous coalitions. No foot with osseous coalition had Stage III arthrosis. The staging severity is associated with the type of the coalition (odds ratio, 7.933; 95% CI, 1.478–42.581; P = .016).

All the patients in this retrospective review had surgery on at least 1 foot for symptomatic middle facet TCC. At the time of submission, 80% of the feet (28 of 35; 95%

Table 2 Coalition type, stage, and age in all patients								
	Osseous and Fibrous			**Osseous**			**Fibrous**	
	Number of Feet	%	Mean Age in Years (Range)	Number of Feet	%	Mean Age in Years (Range)	Number of Feet	%	Mean Age in Years (Range)
Stage I	20	57.1	14 (8–19)	3	30	15 (12–16)	17	68	13 (8–19)
Stage II	12	34.3	25 (10–56)	7	70	29 (10–56)	5	20	20 (10–48)
Stage III	3	8.6	41 (18–56)	0	0	n/a	3	12	41 (18–56)
Total	35	—	20 (8–56)	10	29	24 (10–56)	25	71	17 (8–56)

Abbreviation: n/a, not applicable.

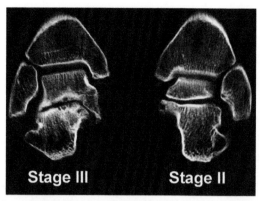

Fig. 3. 56-year-old female with Stage III arthrosis of her right posterior facet and fibrous middle facet coalition with obvious presence of numerous subchondral cysts, subchondral sclerosis, and significant asymmetric posterior facet joint space narrowing. The contralateral side (*left*) has an osseous middle facet TCC (not depicted on this slice) with less severe (Stage II) posterior facet arthrosis.

CI, 63.1%–91.6%) were managed surgically. Of the 28 managed feet surgically, Stage I arthritis was present in 17 (85% of the 20 Stage I feet; 95% CI, 62.1%–96.8%), Stage II in 8 (66.7% of the 12 Stage II feet; 95% CI, 34.9%–90.1%), and Stage III in 3 (100% of the 3 Stage III feet; 95% CI, 29.2%–100%). Of those surgically managed feet, 5 Stage I (29.4%), 2 Stage II (25%), and 3 Stage III (100%) had joint destructive procedures performed.

Of the 35 feet, 25 feet (71.4%; 95% CI, 53.7–85.4%) had fibrous coalitions and 10 feet (28.6%; 95% CI, 14.6–46.3) had osseous coalitions. Of those 25 feet with fibrous coalitions, 17 (68%; 95% CI, 46.5%–85.1%), 5 (20%; 95% CI, 6.8%–40.7%), and 3 (12%; 95% CI, 2.6%–31.2%) had Stage I, II, and III arthrosis, respectively. Of the 10 feet with osseous coalitions, 3 (30%; 95% CI, 6.7%–65.3%), 7 (70%; 95% CI, 34.7%–93.3%), and 0 (0%; 95% CI, 0.0%–30.9%) had Stage I, II, and III arthrosis, respectively. See **Fig. 4** for further clarification.

DISCUSSION

It is important to be able to stage the extent of subtalar joint arthrosis because its presence may dictate whether a fusion should be performed or not. However, no prior study has attempted to grade posterior facet arthrosis objectively, either with plain film radiographs or with CT, in a large surgically managed cohort of patients with middle facet TCC. The CT staging system that the authors developed uses the grading system for hallux rigidus as a template.[14] Based on the literature review presented in this article, it is obvious that the guidelines for determining the need for a fusion are somewhat blurred and a staging system is critically needed.

Kumar and colleagues[6] distinguished between the types of middle facet TCC based on a preoperative CT staging system: osseous, cartilaginous, or fibrous. They did not attempt to grade or quantify the extent or contribution of posterior facet arthrosis in their cohort. They recommend coalition resection in symptomatic cases, regardless of its size relative to the posterior facet in all instances.

Wilde and colleagues[9] used CT with 5-mm slices to evaluate the width of the coalition, the width of the posterior facet of the calcaneus, the cross-sectional area of the coalition relative to the area of the posterior facet, posterior talocalcaneal joint

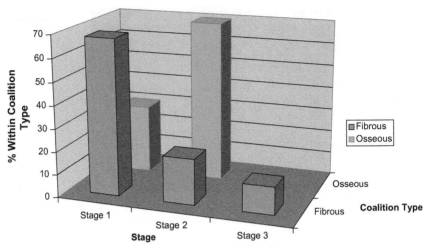

Multinomial Logistic Regression OR = 7.933 (95% CI 1.478 - 42.581), p=0.016

Fig. 4. Arthrosis stage by coalition type.

narrowing, and heel position. They performed 20 middle facet TCC resections in 17 patients.

In their study, the 10 feet with significant heel valgus (>16°) and/or posterior facet joint narrowing had the poorest results of the group, suggesting that heel valgus and/or subtalar arthrosis may be predictors of poor outcomes. Furthermore, on post-operative CT, all the 10 feet with a fair or poor outcome had posterior facet joint space narrowing. Wilde and colleagues[9] concluded that coronal CT is necessary to select feet suitable for resection, although their technique for evaluating posterior facet arthrosis did not scrutinize the posterior facet to the extent that ours does.

Westberry and colleagues[8] used preoperative CT to evaluate for the absence of subtalar joint arthrosis before performing complete resection of the sustentaculum tali in 10 patients with 12 middle facet coalitions. They identified that "there were no cases with evidence of early arthrosis involving the talocalcaneal articulation" in their young patient cohort (mean age of 12.7 years). Westberry's article suggests that the size of the middle facet TCC does not necessarily affect the results of outcome, as the entire sustentaculum tali was excised in their cohort.

Salomao and colleagues[15] studied 22 patients with 32 symptomatic TCCs who were treated with resection and autogenous free fat interposition. Although CT scans were obtained in all cases preoperatively, they did not grade the extent or contribution of subtalar joint arthrosis in their cohort. They concluded that a CT scan should be used in diagnosing TCC, but they did not indicate that it should be used in guiding the surgeon between fusion and resection.

Secondary arthrosis may develop in the rearfoot complex as a result of tarsal coalition, and when present, simple resection alone may not be appropriate.[2,16] Isolated arthrosis of the subtalar joint may occur, and this may best be determined with CT.[10] Scranton[5] suggests that when more than 50% of the subtalar joint is involved, arthrodesis should be performed. When talonavicular joint arthrosis is not present, the senior author (NMB) believes that resection (of the coalition) should be performed in the absence of significant subtalar joint spurring and subchondral cysts with less than 50% posterior facet involvement as seen on CT.[2] Luhmann and Schoenecker[1] demonstrated that a statistically significant poorer outcome was associated with a TCC involving more than 50% of the surface area of the posterior facet identified with CT. But the authors pointed out that 8 of 25 feet with TCC larger than 50% of the posterior facet surface area had good or excellent results, and stated that "TCC size does not absolutely predict postresection outcome."[1] With regard to narrowing of the posterior facet on CT, Wilde and colleagues[9] reported a less optimal result in those feet that did have a narrowed posterior facet. Luhmann and Schoenecker[1] did not find that a narrowed posterior facet had a significant negative effect on short-term outcome. Comfort and Johnson[17] found that good or excellent clinical results were achieved in 77% of 17 coalition resections that involved less than one-third of the entire subtalar joint surface as measured on a coronal CT view.

In our cohort, there was a statistically significant association between patient's age at the time of CT scan and stage of posterior facet arthrosis associated with fibrous and osseous coalition (slope, 0.547; $P = .001$; see earlier discussion). This suggests that arthrosis of the subtalar joint associated with middle facet TCC is a progressive process. It may be beneficial to surgically intervene before the onset of rearfoot arthrosis, especially because one considers a coalition resection or a coalition resection combined with single-stage flat foot reconstruction rather than rearfoot arthrodesis (a joint destructive procedure).[2] An interesting finding of this study is that only the fibrous coalitions were associated with Stage III (end-stage) arthrosis. Because Stage III arthrosis was not present in the osseous group, the authors suggest that an osseous coalition may have a protective effect on the subtalar joint, guarding the joint from developing end-stage arthrosis. Perhaps the theoretical micromotion that may be present at the fibrous middle facet TCC is responsible for the progression to end-stage arthrosis. This suggests that symptomatic osseous coalition may not need to be managed with the same urgency as a fibrous coalition if the goal is to prevent the progression of rearfoot arthrosis. Future prospective studies are the next logical step in evaluating this recommendation.

This CT study demonstrates that varying degrees of arthrosis exist in the subtalar joint when associated with middle facet TCC. When operative intervention was decided for this review spanning 12 years, joint destructive procedures of the subtalar joint were always performed with Stage III arthrosis (100%, 3 of 3 feet), a seemingly obvious appropriate treatment. However, subtalar joint destructive procedures were also performed in a similar percentage of patients with Stage II arthrosis (25%, 2 of 8 feet) and Stage I arthrosis (29.4%, 5 of 17 feet). Although outcomes or indications for surgical intervention were not studied in this retrospective review, theoretically, fewer joint-destructive procedures should be performed in Stage I than in Stage II because less arthrosis exists with a lesser stage. It is unclear as to why any Stage I arthrosis would undergo a joint destructive procedure at all, but it could be performed for significant pes planus or extent of the coalition. However, in recent years, a focus on joint salvage has emerged in conjunction with middle facet TCC treatment, which may not have been considered as a treatment pathway in cases performed earlier in this 12-year review. The authors hope that the CT staging system presented in **Table 1** can be used to compare and contrast future studies, and direct and improve treatment protocols. This use will clarify the current uncertainty about the indications for resection versus arthrodesis strategy.[8]

SUMMARY

Symptomatic middle facet TCC is frequently associated with rearfoot arthrosis that is often managed surgically with rearfoot fusion. However, no objective method for classifying the extent of subtalar joint arthrosis exists. This retrospective CT review presents a staging system for the evaluation of subtalar joint arthrosis associated with middle facet TCC. Most feet (57.1%) exhibited Stage I arthrosis. Stage II arthrosis was present in 12 feet (34.3%), and Stage III arthrosis only in 3 feet (8.6%). The mean age of patients is positively associated with severity, suggesting that early intervention may limit or reduce the progression of subtalar joint arthrosis. Prospective studies are needed to compare the surgical management of symptomatic middle facet TCC more thoroughly. The authors hope that the CT staging system introduced here will assist in comparing the extent of subtalar joint pathology and in incorporating staging in analyses of therapeutic effectiveness.

ACKNOWLEDGMENTS

We thank Howard Barkan, DrPH, for his assistance with statistical analysis.

REFERENCES

1. Luhmann SJ, Schoenecker PL. Symptomatic talocalcaneal coalition resection: indications and results. J Pediatr Orthop 1998;18(6):748–54.
2. Kernbach KJ, Blitz NM, Rush SM. Bilateral single stage middle facet coalition resection combined with flatfoot reconstruction. A report of 3 cases and review of the literature. Investigations involving middle facet coalitions – part I. J Foot Ankle Surg 2008;47(3):180–90.
3. Swiontkowski MF, Scranton PE, Hansen ST. Tarsal coalitions: long-term results of surgical treatment. J Pediatr Orthop 1983;3(3):287–92.
4. Hansen ST. Progressive symptomatic flatfoot (lateral peritalar subluxation). In: Hansen ST, editor. Functional reconstruction of the foot ankle. Philadelphia: Lippincott Williams and Wilkins; 2000. p. 195–7.
5. Scranton PE. Treatment of symptomatic talocalcaneal coalition. J Bone Joint Surg Am 1987;69:533–8.
6. Kumar SJ, Guille JT, Lee MS, et al. Osseous and non-osseous coalition of the middle facet of the talocalcaneal joint. J Bone Joint Surg 1992;74(4):529–35.
7. McCormack TJ, Olney B, Asher M. Talocalcaneal coalition resection: a 10-year follow-up. J Pediatr Orthop 1997;17(1):13–5.
8. Westberry DE, Davids JR, Oros W. Surgical management of symptomatic talocalcaneal coalitions by resection of the sustentaculum tali. J Pediatr Orthop 2003; 23(4):493–7.
9. Wilde PH, Torode IP, Dickens DR, et al. Resection for symptomatic talocalcaneal coalition. J Bone Joint Surg Br 1994;76:797–801.
10. Herzenberg JE, Goldner JL, Martinez S, et al. Computerized tomography of talocalcaneal tarsal coalition: a clinical and anatomic study. Foot Ankle 1986; 6(6):273–88.
11. Saltzman CL, Fehrle MJ, Cooper RR, et al. Triple arthrodesis: twenty-five and forty-four-year follow-up on the same patients. J Bone Joint Surg Am 1999;81: 1391–402.
12. Coester LM, Saltzman CL, Leupold J, et al. Long-term results following ankle arthrodesis for post-traumatic arthritis. J Bone Joint Surg Am 2001;83:219–28.
13. Hosmer DW, Lemeshow S. In Applied logistic regression. 2nd edition. New York: John Wiley and Sons; 1999.
14. Vanore JV, Christensen JC, Kravitz SR, et al. Clinical Practice Guideline First Metatarsophalangeal Joint Disorders Panel of the American College of Foot &

Ankle Surgeons. Diagnosis and treatment of first metatarsophalangeal joint disorders. Section 2: hallux rigidus. J Foot Ankle Surg 2003;42:124–36.

15. Salomão O, Napoli MM, de Carvalho AE, et al. Talocalcaneal coalition: diagnosis and surgical management. Foot Ankle Int 1992;13:251–6.

16. Kernbach KJ, Blitz NM. The presence of calcaneal fibular remodeling associated with middle facet talocalcaneal coalition: a retrospective CT review of 35 feet. Investigations involving middle facet coalitions–Part II. J Foot Ankle Surg 2008; 47(4):288–94.

17. Comfort TK, Johnson L. Resection for symptomatic talocalcaneal coalition. J Pediatr Orthop 1998;18:283–8.

Congenital Vertical Talus: A Review

Janay Mckie, MD[a], Timothy Radomisli, MD[a,b],*

KEYWORDS

- Vertical talus • Convex pes planus
- Flatfoot deformity • Pes planus

Congenital vertical talus (CVT), also known as congenital convex pes valgus, is a severe form of congenital rigid flatfoot. The first complete clinical, radiological, anatomic, and pathologic study was published in 1914 by Mlle R. Henke. CVT is an uncommon disorder defined by rigid dorsal dislocation of the navicular on the talar head and neck. In addition to the irreducible dorsal dislocation of the navicular (type 1 form), this condition can also include deformity of the calcaneocuboid joint (type 2 form). Radiographically observed, the talus is in a vertical position and the navicular is dorsally dislocated when the foot is placed in maximum dorsiflexion and plantar flexion. CVT has an incidence of 1 in 10,000 and affects males and females with equal frequency. Fifty percent of CVT cases present as an isolated (idiopathic) deformity, whereas the other 50% occur in association with neuromuscular or genetic disorders. The cause of this deformity is unknown; however, existing evidence suggests that some isolated deformities are transmitted as an autosomal dominant trait with incomplete penetrance.[1,2]

ETIOLOGY

CVT has been linked with defects of the central nervous system (CNS), muscle abnormalities, acquired deformities, and certain genetic conditions. CNS defects associated with CVT include, but are not limited to, diastematomyelia, lipoma of the cauda equina, myelomeningocele, sacral agenesis, arthrogryposis, and neurofibromatosis. These CNS defects are associated with a more rigid form of vertical talus. This more rigid form is secondary to the associated severe muscle imbalances and the bony dislocation characteristic of CVT. An ischiocalcaneus band is a muscle abnormality also associated with CVT. It is a rare fibrous anlage of muscle that originates from the ischium, spans the popliteal space, and blends distally into the aponeurosis

[a] Department of Orthopaedic Surgery, The Mount Sinai Medical Center, 5 East 98th Street, 9th Floor, New York, NY 10029, USA
[b] Department of Orthopedic Surgery, Lenox Hill Hospital, 130 East 77th Street, 12th Floor, New York, NY 10075, USA
* Corresponding author. Department of Orthopedic Surgery, Lenox Hill Hospital, 130 East 77th Street, 12th Floor, New York, NY 10075.
E-mail address: tradomisli@gmail.com (T. Radomisli).

Clin Podiatr Med Surg 27 (2010) 145–156
doi:10.1016/j.cpm.2009.08.008
0891-8422/09/$ – see front matter © 2010 Elsevier Inc. All rights reserved.

of the triceps surae. In addition to the CVT produced by the contracture of the triceps surae, this muscular abnormality is associated with a flexion contracture of the knee.

Acquired deformities associated with CVT include, but are not limited to, cerebral palsy, polio, and spinal muscular atrophy. CVT can also be precipitated by overcorrection of a clubfoot deformity. Genetic syndromes that include CVT as a part of their clinical spectrum include Patau, Edwards, Freeman-Sheldon, Smith-Lemli-Opitz, nail-patella, Marfan, multiple pterygium, Hurler, de Barsy, and Eagle-Barrett syndromes.

RELEVANT ANATOMY

Multiple pathoanatomical changes occur to varying degrees as a result of CVT. The navicular is displaced onto the dorsolateral aspect of the talar head and neck. This leads to the navicular becoming wedge-shaped with a hypoplastic plantar segment. The talar head is flattened dorsally, and its articular cartilage expands to accommodate the articular surface of the displaced navicular. Within the ankle plafond, only the posterior one-third of the talar dome articulates as the calcaneus is plantarflexed and rotated posterolaterally. The sustenaculum tali is hypoplastic and provides no support to the talar head. The anterior and middle subtalar facets are either absent or replaced by fibrous tissue, and the posterior facet is misshapen with increased lateral tilt. The cuboid is laterally displaced. The plantar half of the cuboid may be hypotrophic when a large degree of dorsal subluxation or frank dislocation occurs through the entire transverse tarsal articulation.

These pathoanatomical changes are accompanied by alterations in the ligaments and muscles. The ligaments on the plantar surface of the talocalcaneonavicular joint are attenuated. The calcaneonavicular (spring) ligament and the anterior fibers of the deltoid ligament are stretched. This stretching includes the medial fibers of the bifurcate ligament. There are contractures of the lateral portions of the dorsal talonavicular, calcaneofibular, interosseous talocalcaneal ligaments, and posterior capsules of the ankle and subtalar joints. The proximal and distal components of the dorsal retinaculum of the ankle merge and are reduced to a thick, shortened structure at the apex of the dorsal deformity, which is in line with the anterior surface of the tibia. The dorsal retinaculum of the ankle becomes fibrotic and acts as a fulcrum, increasing the mechanical advantage of the extensor musculature that passes acutely beneath it and inserts onto the laterally displaced foot. The superior peroneal retinaculum becomes attenuated, leading to the ability of the peroneal tendons to subluxate anteriorly on the fibula.

The triceps surae, tibialis anterior, long toe extensors, and peronei are contracted. The tibialis posterior is subluxated anteriorly, creating a groove in the medial malleolus resulting in the tendon splaying out and becoming attenuated as it passes onto the plantar surface of the midfoot. In addition, the anteriorly subluxated peroneals bowstring across the midfoot. These changes in the course of the tibialis posterior and peroneals results in the muscles becoming dorsiflexor rather than their normal plantarflexor. The triceps surae has a broad insertion onto the superolateral aspect of the tuberosity of the everted calcaneus. If left untreated, all of the aforementioned osseous, muscular, and ligamentous changes may result in a painful, rigid flatfoot with weak push-off power.[3,4]

CLINICAL EVALUATION

Flatfoot is one of the most common conditions seen in the pediatric orthopedic practice. In the evaluation of a patient with flatfoot, the examiner must distinguish between flexible and nonflexible flatfoot deformity. Furthermore, the type of deformity must be categorized by the presence or absence of pain. Determining the specific features associated with flatfoot deformity determines management options: surgical versus nonsurgical. In a newborn presenting with flatfoot deformity, the differential diagnosis includes positional calcaneovalgus deformity of the foot, posteromedial bowing of the tibia, congenital absence of the fibula, congenital oblique talus, idiopathic flat feet, and CVT.[5,6]

Patients with CVT present with a "Persian slipper foot,"[3] a lateral longitudinal column with abducted plantar contour, elongated and convex medial longitudinal column, and elevated and clawed lateral toes (**Fig. 1**). On physical examination, the talus is palpable medially at the sole of the foot (**Fig. 2**). The sole is convex thereby creating the characteristic rocker-bottom deformity (**Fig. 3**). The forefoot is in an abducted and dorsiflexed position. The hindfoot is in equinovalgus.

The rigid flatfoot deformity produced by CVT does not delay walking. The patient with uncorrected CVT will have a peg-leg gait (an awkward gait with limited forefoot push-off) with callus under a prominent talar head. The heel will have no contact with the ground. In fact, weight-bearing occurs on an area that is approximately the size of a half-dollar. The deformity resists manipulation because of the contracted ligaments, capsules, and tendons. Because CVT is seen in frequent association with other underlying primary diagnoses and congenital abnormalities, a thorough search for other congenital and developmental disorders must be performed on initial evaluation of patients presenting with CVT.

RADIOLOGY

In the newborn, only rounded ossific nuclei of some bones of the foot are visible radiographically. Ossification of the hindfoot is confined to the talus and the calcaneus. The calcaneus starts to ossify by week 23 of gestation. The talus starts to ossify at approximately 28 weeks of gestation. The cuboid appears at 6 to 7 months. The navicular takes 9 months to 5 years for ossification to occur. The cuneiforms begin ossification

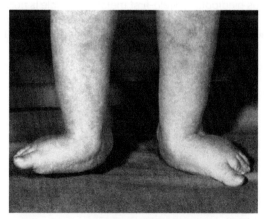

Fig. 1. "Persian slipper foot" illustrated in an 18-month-old child with CVT bilaterally secondary to Freeman-Sheldon syndrome. Note that the heel is non–weight-bearing and the medial longitudinal column is elongated; the foot is elevated, abducted, and pronated. (*From* Drennan JC. Congenital vertical talus. Instr Course Lect 1996;45:315–22; with permission.)

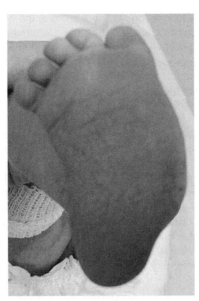

Fig. 2. Plantar aspect of foot of a 6-month-old infant with CVT. Note the fixed forefoot abduction and the medial prominence of the talus. (*Reproduced from* Dobbs MB, Purcell DB, Nunley R, et al. Early results of a new method of treatment for idiopathic congenital vertical talus. J Bone Joint Surg Am 2006;88(6):1192–200; with permission.)

between 3 months and 2.5 years of age, with the lateral cuneiform appearing first. The metatarsals and phalanges are usually present at birth. Female ossification centers appear earlier than male ossification centers.[7]

In evaluating the pediatric foot, several key radiographic angles are necessary. On anterior-posterior radiograph, the talocalcaneal and talo-first metatarsal angle are significant. The talocalcaneal (Kite) angle is normally 20° to 40° in children younger than 5 years.[8] An increased angle results in a valgus hindfoot, whereas a decreased angle results in varus hindfoot. The talo-first metatarsal angle is normally −10° (varus) to +30° (valgus).[8] On lateral radiograph, relevant angles include the talocalcaneal, tibiocalcaneal, tibiotalar, and talo-first metatarsal angles. Of particular importance is

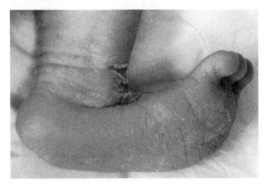

Fig. 3. Characteristic rocker-bottom deformity. Lateral aspect of foot of a 6-month-old infant with congenital vertical talus. Note rigid convex plantar surface. (*Reproduced from* Dobbs MB, Purcell DB, Nunley R, et al. Early results of a new method of treatment for idiopathic congenital vertical talus. J Bone Joint Surg Am 2006;88(6):1192–200; with permission.)

the tibiocalcaneal angle, which normally increases with plantar flexion and decreases with dorsiflexion of the ankle.

In addition to the traditional anterior-posterior and lateral radiographs, dynamic films (radiographic studies done in maximum dorsiflexion/plantar flexion) are essential in the evaluation of the pediatric foot. Significant angles include the talocalcaneal, tibiocalcaneal, and talo-first metatarsal angles. Normally, the talocalcaneal angle is 25° to 55° in dorsiflexion.[8] The tibiocalcaneal angle is normally 25° to 60° in dorsiflexion. Increases in either angle occur in equinus or varus deformities.[8]

CVT must be distinguished radiographically from the more common oblique talus deformity because both present similarly but have distinctly different treatment options. CVT is vertical placement of the talus and rigid talonavicular dislocation, whereas in oblique talus deformity, the talonavicular joint maintains its articulation and is dorsally subluxated in dorsiflexion or standing position. Furthermore, the oblique talus foot is reducible with plantar flexion of the forefoot. At birth, the midfoot is not yet ossified but in CVT, the vertical talus lies parallel to the anatomic axis of the tibia. Also, the calcaneus is in equinus angulation with a dorsiflexed and laterally translated forefoot.

The radiographic evaluation of the pediatric foot is difficult because of limitations in visualizing ossification centers. However, there are characteristic soft-tissue radiographic findings that can be appreciated in the newborn period as it relates to CVT. An example of this would be the distinct plantar surface convexity, also described as rocker-bottom deformity. This information plus bony deformity can be used to diagnose CVT. Workup of CVT includes anterior-posterior, lateral, and dynamic films. The anterior-posterior view will show an increased talocalcaneal angle because of the equinovalgus angulation of the os calcis. On the lateral view, the talo-horizontal and tibiotalar angles approach 90° and 180°, respectively. On dynamic views, the maximally dorsiflexed view will show a rigidly fixed hindfoot equinus. The maximally plantarflexed view will show irreducibility of the midfoot on the hindfoot (**Fig. 4**). This finding on dynamic view helps to make the definitive diagnosis of CVT.

Of the other imaging modalities, magnetic resonance imaging provides a clear outline of the cartilaginous anlage of bones; however, its use is currently limited to research applications.[3] It has also been used to assess the presence of intrinsic and extrinsic muscles that may create an imbalance leading to the development of CVT.

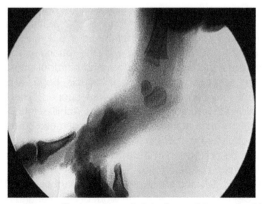

Fig. 4. Maximum stress plantar flexion view of right foot of 2-month-old male infant. Note irreducibility of the midfoot on the hindfoot, diagnostic of CVT.

TREATMENT

Restoration of the normal anatomic relationships between the bones of the foot and reestablishment of the weight-bearing capacity of the first ray are the goals of treating this severely rigid foot deformity. Because CVT presents in varying degrees of deformity and severity, various operative approaches have been described. For example, patients with neuromuscular or neural tube defects tend to have more rigid deformities that require muscle-balancing procedures.

Closed treatment with manipulation and casting was the earliest technique used for CVT management. Through years of clinical experience, surgeons have learned that serial casting alone does not resolve CVT. Jacobsen and Crawford's 1983 literature survey[9] of 273 patients with CVT who were treated with the Coleman-Stelling technique determined that surgically treated patients fared better than those treated nonoperatively. The current standard is that serial casting be used primarily as initial treatment to supplement surgery. Casting achieves the objective of stretching the foot in plantar flexion and inversion while counterpressure is applied to the medial aspect of the talus. Elongating and stretching the talonavicular joint facilitates its reduction. This is an important step in avoiding compression of the dorsally displaced navicular into the talus. Casts are usually changed every 1 to 2 weeks.

Since 1914, when CVT was first described as an entity, treatment has evolved from solely nonsurgical to combined nonsurgical and surgical techniques. In general, any surgical intervention is usually delayed until the child is about 12 to 18 months old. Better surgical prognosis depends on how early surgery is done. In 1939, Lamy and Weissman[10] recommended excision of the talus for definitive treatment of this rigid flatfoot deformity. In 1967, Eyre-Brooke[11] advocated excising the navicular. Today, neither of these techniques is accepted as definitive treatment.

Osmond-Clarke[12] (1956), Herndon and Heyman[13] (1963), and Coleman and colleagues[14] (1970) described a staged, two-incision reconstructive surgery. According to Coleman, stage 1 involved lengthening of the extensor digitorum longus, extensor hallucis longus, and tibialis anterior, with capsulotomies of the talonavicular and calcaneocuboid joints. This stage also included a release of the talocalcaneal interosseous ligament. The second stage involved tendo-Achilles lengthening with a posterior capsulotomy of the ankle and subtalar joints.

In 1979, Ogata and colleagues[1] recommended a single-stage procedure with medial approach, after noting the high incidence of complications with the two-stage technique. In 1987, Seimon[15] described a single-stage dorsal approach. "Surgical correction of congenital vertical talus under the age of 2 years," describes the evaluation of 7 patients (10 feet) with an average follow-up of 5.2 years. Seimon suggested that the pathomechanics of CVT correlated with the rationale of surgical treatment. Therefore, treatment must correct both forefoot and hindfoot deformities. In the Seimon approach (dorsal approach), the extensor hallucis longus and peroneus tertius were tenotomized and the talonavicular joint was opened. The talonavicular joint was reduced and held with a Kirschner wire and the Achilles tendon was lengthened percutaneously. This approach resulted in excellent cosmetic correction in 7 feet and good cosmetic correction in 3 feet. Seimon and colleagues concluded that there was no need for surgery to be performed in 2 stages. Furthermore, extensive surgery was not necessary for correction of deformity.

Stricker and Rosen[16] (1997) and Mazzocca and colleagues[17] (2001) published their experience with the Seimon technique. In the work of Stricker and Rosen, 13 patients (20 feet) were evaluated. The outcome was evaluated by a scoring system of 7 clinical and 8 radiographic parameters to determine correction of all feet at an average follow-up of 41 months. Seventeen feet had good results and 3 had fair results. Clinically, some patients occasionally experienced postoperative stiffness of ankle and subtalar motion. Radiographically, many feet were seen to have mild residual forefoot abduction with midfoot sagging at the talonavicular joint. Overall, Stricker and Rosen had success with the Seimon technique. They concluded that this single-stage technique resulted in good correction with plantigrade, painless feet, particularly in patients younger than 27 months.

Mazzocca and colleagues retrospectively compared the single-stage dorsal approach (Seimon approach) and the posterior approach to treating CVT. Twenty-four patients (33 feet) treated between 1960 and 1998 were evaluated.[17] Group one, 18 patients (25 feet), consisted of feet treated with the posterior approach, a multiple-incision technique. Group two, 6 patients (18 feet), consisted of feet treated with the dorsal approach with a single incision made dorsally in the transverse-oblique orientation over the anterior inferior ankle crease, from the talonavicular joint laterally to the tip of the fibula. There was a minimal 3-year follow-up with evaluation of preoperative and follow-up radiographs. In addition, postoperative clinical evaluation was achieved via the Adelaar clinical score (**Table 1**). The dorsal approach group had no repeated or revision operations compared with the posterior approach group (45 procedures on 25 feet). Clinically, the dorsal approach group had higher (8.0 vs 6.75) Adelaar clinical scores. Tourniquet time for the posterior approach and dorsal approach group was 123 minutes and 87 minutes, respectively. Complications occurred in 12 patients treated with the posterior approach who developed avascular necrosis (AVN), whereas no patient treated with the dorsal approach had any reported AVN. Both groups had similar preoperative and postoperative radiographic measures. Mazzocca and colleagues concluded that both procedures were able to successfully reduce the talonavicular joint, but the single-stage dorsal incision approach required significantly less operative time, had better clinical scores, and had fewer complications 3 years after surgery.

In 1999, Kodros and Dias[18] described a single-stage approach with a Cincinnati incision, an incision made from the medial cuneiform to the lateral malleolus that can be extended to the calcaneocuboid joint. In their work "Single-staged surgical correction of congenital vertical talus," 41 patients (55 feet) with CVT from various causes were evaluated: 30 feet with associated neural tube defects, 10 feet with neuromuscular disorders, 5 feet with congenital malformation syndromes, and 10 feet with idiopathic CVT. All feet were treated with the single-stage surgical correction

Table 1	
Adelaar-Williams-Gould scoring system for CVT	
Clinical appearance	• Poor cosmetic appearance
	• Ankle and subtalar motion loss
	• Prominent talar head
	• Loss of medial longitudinal arch
	• Hindfoot valgus
	• Abnormal shoe wear
Radiographic appearance (weight-bearing)	• Abnormal talonavicular angle
	• Hindfoot equinus
	• Talar metatarsal axis
	• Talonavicular subluxation

Key: Each clinical and radiographic criterion is worth 1 point. For each criterion, subtract 1 point from 10 to get the score.

via Cincinnati incision by a single surgeon. Thirty-two patients (42 feet) were available for clinical and radiographic follow-up, averaging 7 years from the time of surgery. Over this period of time, there were no wound complications or AVN of the talus. Ten feet needed reoperation. At final follow-up, there were 31 good and 11 fair clinical and radiographic outcomes. Radiographically evaluated, there was improvement in the anterior-posterior and lateral talocalcaneal and talo-first metatarsal angles, which were within the range of normal angles.

In 2006, Dobbs and colleagues[19] advocated even less surgery for CVT than was previously proposed by other investigators. Their approach to CVT involved a combination of casting, percutaneous Kirchner wire pinning of the talonavicular joint, and percutaneous heel-cord tenotomy. In their study, the goal was to evaluate a new method of manipulation and cast immobilization, based on principles used by Ponseti for the treatment of clubfoot deformity, followed by pinning of the talonavicular joint and percutaneous tenotomy of the Achilles tendon (**Figs. 5–7**). Dobbs and colleagues noted that the traditional treatment method for CVT, involving manipulation and application of a cast followed by extensive soft-tissue releases, was often followed by severe stiffness of the foot and other complications. These complications included wound necrosis, talar necrosis, undercorrection of the deformity, stiffness in the ankle and subtalar joint, pseudoarthrosis, and the eventual need for multiple operative procedures (eg, subtalar and triple arthrodesis).

In their study, Dobbs and colleagues clinically and radiographically evaluated 11 patients (19 feet) at the time of presentation, immediately after surgery, and at the time of latest follow-up. Casting was done in a technique similar to those used by Ponseti to correct a clubfoot deformity, but with the forces applied in the opposite direction. Minimal surgery consisting of percutaneous Achilles tenotomy (19 feet), fractional lengthening of the anterior tibial tendon (2 feet) or peroneal brevis tendon (1 foot), and percutaneous pin fixation of the talonavicular joint (12 feet) was done. With this minimally invasive correction technique, initial correction was achieved in all 19 feet clinically and radiographically. Five casts were required for correction. No patient underwent any type of extensive surgical releases. Mean ankle dorsiflexion and plantar flexion at final evaluation was 25° and 33°, respectively. Dorsal subluxation

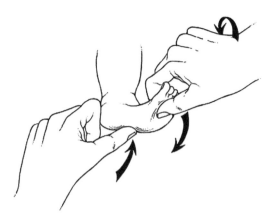

Fig. 5. The manipulative forces necessary to correct vertical talus deformity. The foot is stretched into plantar flexion and inversion while counter pressure is applied to the medial aspect of the head of the talus. (*Reproduced from* Dobbs MB, Purcell DB, Nunley R, et al. Early results of a new method of treatment for idiopathic congenital vertical talus. J Bone Joint Surg Am 2006;88(6):1192–200; with permission.)

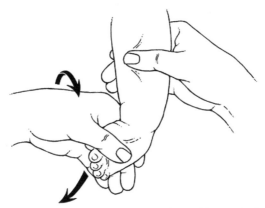

Fig. 6. The foot in maximum hindfoot varus and forefoot adduction before pinning of talo-navicular joint and lengthening of Achilles tendon. (*Reproduced from* Dobbs MB, Purcell DB, Nunley R, et al. Early results of a new method of treatment for idiopathic congenital vertical talus. J Bone Joint Surg Am 2006;88(6):1192–200; with permission.)

of the navicular recurred in 3 patients. At latest follow-up, there was statistically significant improvement in all the measured radiographic parameters compared with pretreatment. Moreover, all of the measured angles were within normal values for patient age. Dobbs and colleagues concluded that serial manipulation and cast immobilization followed by talonavicular pin fixation and percutaneous tenotomy of the Achilles provides excellent results in clinical appearance of the foot, function of the foot, and correction of deformity as measured radiographically at a minimum of 2 years.

Historically various surgical methods have been used to treat CVT. Three basic themes of treatment are apparent on review of the literature exploring CVT: (1) staged multiple-incision technique with extensive soft-tissue release, (2) single-stage medial and posterior approach and single-stage dorsal approach, and (3) minimally invasive technique with casting. The Seimon approach is the most popular intervention used. However, the Dobbs approach of a minimally invasive surgery seems to be another

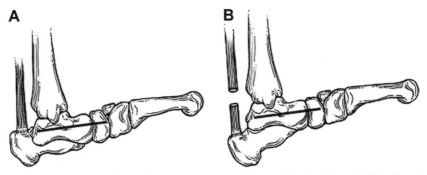

Fig. 7. The minor surgical procedure to correct CVT proposed by Dobbs et al: (*A*) talonavicular reduction with pin but residual equinus; (*B*) percutaneous tenotomy of Achilles tendon that corrects equinus of calcaneus. (*Reproduced from* Dobbs MB, Purcell DB, Nunley R, et al. Early results of a new method of treatment for idiopathic congenital vertical talus. J Bone Joint Surg Am 2006;88(6):1192–200; with permission.)

viable option, but it is limited by its lack of results 2 years after surgery. In general, surgical treatment of CVT is best done in one stage (**Figs. 8** and **9**).

Postoperatively, a patient should be immobilized in a walking short-leg cast after fixation is achieved. In the dorsal approach, the Kirschner wire is retained for 8 weeks and then a walking short leg cast is used for 2 to 4 weeks. In the case of CVT deformity treated via the Cincinnati incision, the foot is immobilized in a plaster cast with wires retained for 4 months. Afterwards, a rigid ankle-foot orthosis is used for long-term support. In terms of future follow-up, typically, patients with idiopathic CVT do not need a postoperative brace or orthosis. However, postoperative bracing is advised for children with myelodysplasia, arthrogryposis, and other syndromes.

As with any operative procedure, treatment of CVT is not without complications in the perioperative, early postoperative, and late postoperative periods. Not unique to CVT are the common perioperative complications of infection, wound-healing problems, and skin slough. In the early postoperative period, deformity can recur. According to Stricker and Rosen, this is usually secondary to undercorrection because of incomplete talonavicular reduction, insufficient posterior ankle release, or residual

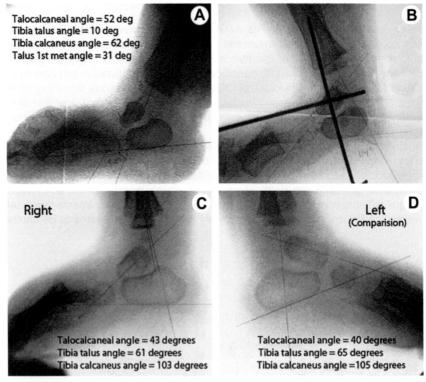

Fig. 8. (A) Preoperative lateral view of right foot of a 7-month-old male infant. (B) Immediate postoperative lateral view of right foot of a 7-month-old male infant. Technique used was the single-stage Cincinnati approach with pantalar release. Note the following angle values: talocalcaneal angle, 46°; tibia talus angle, 68°; tibia calcaneus angle, 114°; talo-first metatarsal angle, 12°. (C, D) Comparative lateral foot views of an 11-month-old male infant, approximately 5-month status post CVT operation (right foot, in C) versus normal nonoperative foot (left foot, in D). The radiographic angles of the operative foot have returned to normal and similar to the patients contralateral unaffected foot.

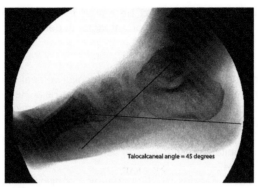

Talocalcaneal angle = 45 degrees

Fig. 9. Lateral fluoroscopic image demonstrating normalized talocalcaneal angle in a 4-year-old boy, status 41 months after single-stage CVT reconstruction.

foot abduction.[16] According to Kodros and Dias, recurrence can also be attributed to neurologic causes. They noted higher rates in patients with spina bifida.[17] For recurrent deformity, salvage procedures include subtalar arthrodesis (Grice-Green procedure), triple arthrodesis, and talectomy. The Grice-Green procedure is used in the case of recurrence in an older child. Triple arthrodesis is reserved for a symptomatic adolescent foot. Talectomy is done in patients with severe, recalcitrant deformities.[9,15,20–22]

Another early postoperative complication of CVT surgery is AVN of the talus. This was a frequent complication of the two-stage release and extensive surgery approach; however, this type of complication is now rare. Works by Kodros and Dias, Seimon, Stricker and Rosen, and Mazzocca and colleagues[16–18] that have used a single-stage approach have not reported occurrences of talar AVN. Late complications of CVT surgery include restricted range of motion of the foot and ankle, which may contribute to calf muscle atrophy and possibly lead to easy fatigue of the affected limb.

With regard to the overall outcome and prognosis of surgically managed CVT, it seems that most patients do well. Some minor calf atrophy and foot size asymmetry may occur. These outcomes usually occur among unilateral cases of CVT. Ankle range of motion is usually about 75% of normal. In those rare occasions in which AVN occur, results are less optimal secondary to ankle pain, stiffness, and weakness.

SUMMARY

The surgical treatment of CVT is evolving and directed toward minimizing the amount of dissection. The benefits appear to be decreasing the risk of AVN and postoperative pain and stiffness. In addition, as awareness of CVT increases amongst the medical community and the general population, early diagnosis and surgical correction in infants younger than 2 years may be achieved. Older children tend to have less favorable results because the original CVT deformity is compounded by unchecked growth of the talar head and neck. This makes the medial longitudinal column excessively long. Deformity in this case may require excision of the navicular to equalize the lengths of the medial and lateral columns.

From the literature review detailing the history of treatment patterns, it is apparent that controversy exists over the type of surgical approaches used to treat CVT. However, choosing which structures to release should be the most important aspect of surgical treatment. Attention should be drawn to the dorsal and dorsolateral contracted tissues. This is the most important factor in determining outcome.

REFERENCES

1. Ogata K, Schoenecker PL, Sheridan J. Congenital vertical talus and its familial occurrence: an analysis of 36 patients. Clin Orthop Relat Res 1979;139:128–32.
2. Dobbs MB, Schoenecker PL, Gordon JE. Autosomal dominant transmission of isolated congenital vertical talus. Iowa Orthop J 2002;22:25–7.
3. Drennan JC. Congenital vertical talus. Instr Course Lect 1995;45:315–22.
4. Specht EE. Congenital paralytic vertical talus: an anatomical study. J Bone Joint Surg Am 1975;57:842–7.
5. Sankar WN, Weiss J, Skaggs DL. Orthopaedic conditions in the newborn. J Am Acad Orthop Surg 2009;17(2):112–22.
6. Sullivan JA. Pediatric flatfoot: evaluation and management. J Am Acad Orthop Surg 1999;7(1):44–53.
7. Katz MA, Davidson RS, Chan PS, et al. Plain radiographic evaluation of the pediatric foot and its deformities. University of Pennsylvania Orthopaedic 1997; 10:30–9.
8. VanderWilde R, Staheli LT, Chew DE, et al. Measurements on radiographs of the foot in normal infants and children. J Bone Joint Surg Am 1988;70:407–15.
9. Jacobsen ST, Crawford AH. Congenital vertical talus. J Pediatr Orthop 1983;3(3): 306–10.
10. Lamy L, Weissman L. Congenital convex pes planus. J Bone Joint Surg 1939;21: 79–91.
11. Eyre-Brook AL. Congenital vertical talus. J Bone Joint Surg Br 1967;49(4):618–27.
12. Osmond-Clarke H. Congenital vertical talus. J Bone Joint Surg Br 1956;38(1): 334–41.
13. Herndon CH, Heyman CH. Problems in the recognition and treatment of congenital pes valgus. J Bone Joint Surg Am 1963;45:413–29.
14. Coleman SS, Stelling FH 3rd, Jarrett J. Pathomechanics and treatment of congenital vertical talus. Clin Orthop Relat Res 1970;70:62–72.
15. Seimon LP. Surgical correction of congenital vertical talus under the age of 2 years. J Pediatr Orthop 1987;7(4):405–11.
16. Stricker SJ, Rosen E. Early one-stage reconstruction of congenital vertical talus. Foot Ankle Int 1997;18(9):535–43.
17. Mazzocca AD, Thomson JD, Deluca PA. Comparison of the posterior approach versus the dorsal approach in the treatment of congenital vertical talus. J Pediatr Orthop 2001;21(2):212–7.
18. Kodros SA, Dias LS. Single-stage surgical correction of congenital vertical talus. J Pediatr Orthop 1999;19(1):42–8.
19. Dobbs MB, Purcell DB, Nunley R, et al. Early results of a new method of treatment for idiopathic congenital vertical talus. J Bone Joint Surg Am 2006;88(6): 1192–200.
20. Dodge LD, Ashley RK, Gilbert RJ. Treatment of the congenital vertical talus: a retrospective review of 36 feet with long-term follow-up. Foot Ankle 1987;7(6): 326–32.
21. Duncan RD, Fixsen JA. Congenital convex pes valgus. J Bone Joint Surg Br 1999;81(2):250–4.
22. Napiontek. Congenital vertical talus: a retrospective and critical review of 32 feet operated on by peritalar reduction. J Pediatr Orthop B 1995;4(2):179–87.

Current Concepts and Techniques
in Foot and Ankle Surgery

Adamantinoma of the Tibia Mimicking a Benign Cystic Lesion: A Case Report

Andreas F. Mavrogenis, MD[a], Spyridon Galanakos, MD[b],
Olga D. Savvidou, MD[c], Panayiotis J. Papagelopoulos, MD, DSc[a],*

KEYWORDS

• Bone tumors • Tibia • Adamantinoma • Cystic lesions • Ankle

Adamantinoma of the long bones is a rare primary malignant bone tumor that is usually located in the diaphysis and less frequently in the metaphysis, with a predilection for the anterior cortex of the tibia (90%). Less common location sites were reported in the ribs, radius, fibula, spine, metatarsal bones, olecranon, and the humerus.[1–8] Fibular involvement is rare but when it does occur, most adamantinomas also involve the adjacent tibia through direct extension, or synchronous or metachronous presentation.[1,2,7]

The histogenesis of adamantinoma is still unknown. The presence of epithelial,[2,9,10] endothelial,[11,12] and synovial cells[13] were implicated as the cells of origin. However, various molecular and cytogenetic studies were unable to identify a consistent and nonrandom cytogenetic aberration.[14–16]

The most common clinical findings of adamantinoma include a dull, insidious, and aching pain of the affected lower extremity with concomitant swelling and deformity or pathologic fractures. Typical imaging findings include a heterogenous osteolytic lesion involving the anterior tibial cortex with multiple, sharply circumscribed lucent zones of various sizes, sclerotic bone surroundings, interspersing between, and extending above and below the lucent zones of the thinning and bulging cortex. Advanced or recurrent adamantinomas may be associated with destruction of the cortex and soft tissue extension.[1,6]

[a] First Department of Orthopaedics, Attikon University General Hospital, Athens University Medical School, 15 Neapoleos Street, 15123 Amarousio, Athens, Greece
[b] Fourth Department of Orthopaedics, KAT General Hospital, 14-16 Trikalon Street, 11526 Ampelokipi, Athens, Greece
[c] Department of Orthopaedics, Thriasio Hospital, Elefsina, 4 Riga Ferreou, Ag. Paraskevi 15342, Athens, Greece
* Corresponding author.
E-mail address: pjp@hol.gr (P. J. Papagelopoulos).

Clin Podiatr Med Surg 27 (2010) 157–165
doi:10.1016/j.cpm.2009.09.003   podiatric.theclinics.com

CASE REPORT

A 29-year-old man presented to the authors' institution with left distal tibia and ankle pain. The patient denied any history of trauma or injury. Medical and social histories were unremarkable. The physical examination was otherwise unremarkable except for the left lower extremity tenderness without any palpable soft tissue mass. No palpable lymph nodes were identified. The overlying skin and neurovascular status were also normal. The range of motion of the left ankle was painful at maximum dorsiflexion and plantar flexion. Routine laboratory analysis including complete blood cell count, serum chemistry, erythrocyte sedimentation rate, and C-reactive protein were within normal limits.

Radiographic findings of the left distal tibia and ankle showed an expansile osteolytic lesion involving the posterior tibial cortex (**Fig. 1**). A computed tomography (CT) scan of the left leg showed a homogeneous, cystic, expansile osteolytic lesion within the tibia with thinning and destruction of the posterior-lateral tibial cortex (**Fig. 2**). Magnetic resonance imaging (MRI) showed a 5.8 × 2.0 × 2.0-cm homogeneous intramedullary lesion of the distal tibia. The lesion showed low-signal intensity in T1-weighted images and high-signal intensity in T2-weighted images (**Fig. 3**). Bone scintigraphy showed increased radioisotope uptake at the distal tibia with no other sites of increased uptake. Trephine bone biopsy was then performed, and histologic examination showed loose clusters of epithelial cells with basaloid and squamous components intermixed within a fibrous stromal tissue. These findings were most consistent with the diagnosis of tibial adamantinoma (**Fig. 4**).

Surgical correction of the deformity and resection of the bone tumor was then performed through a posteromedial approach to the left distal lower extremity. An en bloc

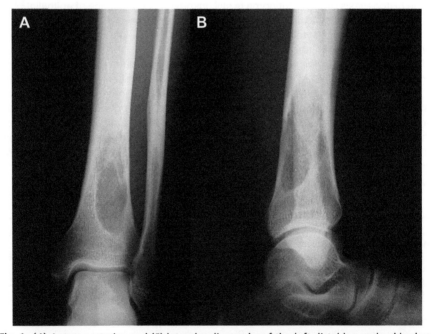

Fig. 1. (*A*) Anteroposterior and (*B*) lateral radiographs of the left distal leg and ankle show a homogeneous expansile osteolytic lesion involving the posterior cortex of the left distal tibia.

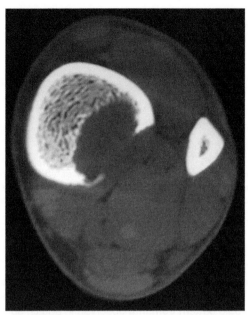

Fig. 2. Axial CT scan of the left leg shows a homogeneous, cystic, expansile osteolytic lesion within the tibia, with thinning and destruction of the posterior-lateral tibial cortex.

resection of the distal third of the tibia was performed, which included the surrounding soft tissues and the fibula. Reconstruction of the bone defect was made by using a 17-cm distal tibia fresh frozen allograft that was fixated to the talus with 3 cancellous screws, and proximally to the host bone with a 9-hole dynamic compression plate and 8 bicortical screws (**Fig. 5**).

The postoperative course was uneventful, and the patient remained nonweight bearing for the first 3 months, followed by partial-weight bearing in a short leg cast for 3 more months. At 4 years' follow-up, there was no evidence of local recurrence or distant metastasis. Imaging studies showed union of the allograft to the host bone (**Fig. 6**).

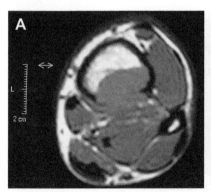
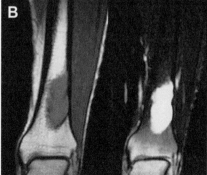

Fig. 3. (*A*) Axial T1-weighted MRI of the left distal tibia shows a homogeneous low-signal intensity lesion within the tibia. (*B*) Coronal T1-weighted (*left*) and T2-weighted (*right*) magnetic resonance images show a homogeneous, low- and high-signal intensity distal tibia lesion, respectively.

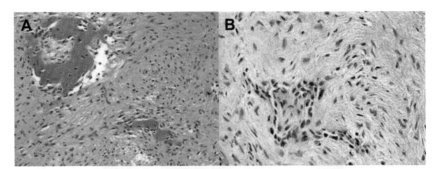

Fig. 4. (*A*) Low-power histologic section shows islands of epithelial cells surrounded by fibrous tissue. (*B*) High-power histologic section shows loose clusters of epithelial cells with basaloid and squamous components intermixed within a fibrous stromal tissue. These findings are consistent with the histologic diagnosis of adamantinoma.

DISCUSSION

Adamantinomas are usually diagnosed after skeletal maturity, most commonly between the ages of 20 and 60, with a slight predilection and a more aggressive course in men.[1,12,17–21] Adamantinomas have also been reported in children, but with a different histologic pattern from that observed in adults, somewhat resembling the histologic pattern of osteofibrous dysplasia defects.[22] The usual pattern of adamantinomas in children was termed differentiated adamantinoma, and usually follows a benign natural course with a favorable prognosis and outcome,[23] or may be the precursor lesion of the classic adamantinoma.[22]

The diaphysis of the tibia is the most common site of extragnathic presentation of adamantinomas. Adamantinomas of the mandible, named ameloblastomas, have similar histologic appearance to the tibial adamantinomas. Ameloblastomas are usually cystic; however, the 2 entities have no other clinical relationship.[24–26]

In early stages, adamantinoma appears as a heterogeneous elongated expansile lucency on plain radiographs, and no periosteal reaction is noted in the surrounding bone. In later stages, a lytic central core with multiple sharply circumscribed lucent zones of various sizes and cortical sclerosis with bulging of the anterior cortex is

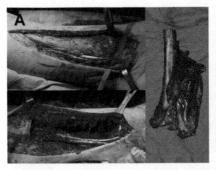
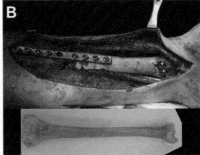

Fig. 5. (*A*) Through the posteromedial approach to the distal leg, en bloc resection of the distal third of the tibia including the surrounding soft tissues and the fibula was done. (*B*) Reconstruction of the bone defect was done using a 17-cm distal tibia fresh frozen allograft that was fixed to the talus with 3 cancellous screws, and proximally to the host bone with a 9-hole dynamic compression plate and 8 bicortical screws.

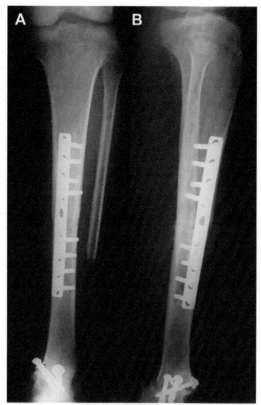

Fig. 6. (*A*) Anteroposterior and (*B*) lateral radiographs of the left leg at 4 years postoperatively show proximal and distal union of the allograft.

apparent. Advanced and recurrent lesions eventually cause cortical thinning and destruction, and soft tissue extension.[6,27,28] CT reveals the heterogeneous osteolytic lesion with expansion and destruction of the cortex, and probable extension to the surrounding soft tissues.[6,28] MRI is useful in differentiating adamantinomas from other bone lesions, such as osteofibrous dysplasia, osteosarcomas, or Ewing sarcomas.[27–29] T1-weighted MRI shows a low-signal intensity heterogeneous lesion, whereas T2-weighted imaging shows a brighter signal that does not diminish with the fat suppression technique.[1]

A bone biopsy of the lytic lesion should be obtained for the accurate diagnosis of these lytic lesions. The microscopic appearance of adamantinoma shows a wide range of morphologic patterns, which can mimic many primary or metastatic bone tumors.[6] Two distinct cellular components are consistently found in histologic specimens but not with enough evidence to suggest an epithelial or biphasic (both epithelial and mesenchymal) origin of the tumor.[9,10,18,21] Four epithelioid histologic patterns have been described: the basaloid type, with cords and islands of cells similar to basal cell carcinoma; the spindle cellular type, similar to the basaloid, but with no peripheral palisading layer; the tubular type, with small ramified tubules or alveolar cavities, matted by 1 or more layers of cubic-cylindrical cells; and the squamous cellular type, with nodules of squamous cells. It is usual for more than 1 type to coexist in the same tumor.[6,19,30] The mesenchymal (fibrous) component of the tumor is composed of a loose arrangement of immature spindle cells producing wisps of collagen. The cells are of a variety of sizes and shapes, and the stellate shape of the nuclei closely resembles that of the primitive dysplastic mesenchymal cells that also make up the stroma of fibrous dysplasia bone defects.[9,10,18,21]

Recent studies based on DNA flow and image cytometry, p53 immunohistochemistry, and immunohistochemical studies in the expression of fibroblast growth factor type 2 (FGF-2), epidermal growth factor and their respective receptors FGFR-1 and EGFR, and the proliferation marker Ki-67 have indicated that cells with an epithelial phenotype are most probably the malignant element of the tumor.[15,16,27,31,32]

The treatment of choice for adamantinomas of the long bones is wide excision by amputation[12,20,33] or limb salvage surgery.[1,30,31,34] Treatment options currently available for reconstruction following limb salvage surgery include the use of an autograft, allograft or endoprosthesis reconstruction,[35–44] and bone transport through the Ilizarov apparatus.[45]

There is a consensus that bone autografts should be predominantly used in children and upper extremity reconstructions following limb salvage surgery.[36,37] The use of vascularized fibula grafts is attractive but, in practice, while bone union usually takes place, hypertrophy of the graft sufficient to allow full weight bearing can take up to 2 years, which is a major disadvantage especially for cancer patients.[40,46] In addition, the longer the segment to be replaced, the higher the incidence of complications.[40]

The combination of a vascularized fibula graft with an allograft is considered the treatment of choice for reconstruction after limb salvage surgery for sarcomas of the tibia.[47] In the femur, however, numerous studies have outlined the risk for complications that occur within the first 2 to 3 years following allograft surgery.[48–53] These complications include an infection rate of 18.5% to 30%,[48,49] a delayed union or nonunion rate of 30% to 63%,[48,53] and an allograft fracture rate of 19% to 42%,[50,51] and may necessitate additional procedures in a significant number of patients.[49,54] In addition, nonweight bearing and protective weight bearing is necessary for up to 16 months until allograft-host bone union.[52] Moreover, the immunosuppressive effect of chemotherapy and radiation therapy and the increased complication rates associated with these treatment options in cancer patients following limb salvage surgery is well documented.[48,49,51,55]

The use of segmental endoprostheses is associated with fewer complication rates, excellent functional results with preserved function of the adjacent joints, and early weight bearing and return to daily activities.[41–43] However, one of the challenges of diaphyseal endoprostheses is the risk of late failure, which has been reported up to 63% at 10 years.[41]

Adamantinomas are highly radioresistant,[56] and chemotherapy has not been shown to be effective.[19,57] The propensity of adamantinomas for metastasis and local recurrence is limited. The rate of metastasis reported in the literature is approximately 15% to 30%.[2,19,20] The tumor usually metastasizes to the lungs, the regional lymph nodes, or the bones.[8,58] Rare pleuropulmonary manifestations, such as hemoptysis, pneumothorax,[6,59] severe paraneoplastic, humorally mediated hypercalcemia, hypercalcemic coma, and pancreatitis have also been reported.[58]

SUMMARY

In this article the imaging findings, diagnosis, and treatment of a patient with a distal tibial adamantinoma presenting as a cystic lesion is presented. The current case shows that adamantinoma may masquerade as a benign bone lesion, but the imaging studies of the distal tibia were highly suggestive of a cystic lesion. The typical location and clinical features, the hazard of a pathologic fracture, and the need for definitive diagnosis and treatment led to prompt biopsy, histopathological diagnosis, and adequate treatment.

REFERENCES

1. Unni KK. Dahlin's bone tumors: general aspects and data on 11,087 cases. 5th edition. Philadelphia: Lippincott-Raven; 1996. p. 333–42.
2. Keeney GL, Unni KK, Beabout JW, et al. Adamantinoma of long bones. A clinico-pathologic study of 85 cases. Cancer 1989;64(3):730–7.
3. Beppu H, Yamaguchi H, Yoshimura N, et al. Adamantinoma of the rib metasta-sizing to the liver. Intern Med 1994;33(7):441–5.
4. Bourne MH, Wood MB, Shives TC. Adamantinoma of the radius: a case report. Orthopedics 1988;11(11):1565–6.
5. Clarke RP, Leonard JR, von Kuster L, et al. Adamantinoma of the humerus with early metastases and death: a case report with autopsy findings. Orthopedics 1989;12(8):1121–5.
6. Filippou DK, Papadopoulos V, Kiparidou E, et al. Adamantinoma of tibia: a case of late local recurrence along with lung metastases. J Postgrad Med 2003;49(1): 75–7.
7. Mohler DG, Cunningham DC. Adamantinoma arising in the distal fibula treated with distal fibulectomy: a case report and review of the literature. Foot Ankle Int 1997;18(11):746–51.
8. Soucacos PN, Hartofilakidis GK, Touliatos AS, et al. Adamantinoma of the olec-ranon. A report of a case with serial metastasizing lesions. Clin Orthop Relat Res 1995;310:194–9.
9. Hazelbag HM, Fleuren GJ, van den Broek LJ, et al. Adamantinoma of the long bones: keratin subclass immunoreactivity pattern with reference to its histogen-esis. Am J Surg Pathol 1993;17(12):1225–33.
10. Rosai J, Pinkus GS. Immunohistochemical demonstration of epithelial differentia-tion in adamantinoma of the tibia. Am J Surg Pathol 1982;6(5):427–34.
11. Changus GW, Speed JS, Stewart FW. Malignant angioblastoma of bone. A reap-praisal of adamantinoma of long bone. Cancer 1957;20(3):540–59.
12. Huvos AG, Marcove RC. Adamantinoma of long bones. A clinicopathological study of fourteen cases with vascular origin suggested. J Bone Joint Surg Am 1975;57(2):148–54.
13. Hicks JD. Synovial sarcoma of the tibia. J Pathol Bacteriol 1954;67(1):151–61.
14. Bridge JA, Dembinski A, DeBoer J, et al. Clonal chromosomal abnormalities in osteofibrous dysplasia. Implications for histopathogenesis and its relationship with adamantinoma. Cancer 1994;73(6):1746–52.
15. Hazelbag HM, Fleuren GJ, Cornelisse CJ, et al. DNA aberrations in the epithelial cell component of adamantinoma of long bones. Am J Pathol 1995;147(6): 1770–9.
16. Hazelbag HM, Wessels JW, Mollevangers P, et al. Cytogenetic analysis of ada-mantinoma of long bones: further indications for a common histogenesis with os-teofibrous dysplasia. Cancer Genet Cytogenet 1996;97(1):5–11.
17. Campanacci M. Adamantinoma of the long bones. Bone and soft tissue tumors. New York: Springer; 1990. p. 629–38.
18. Hauben E, van den Broek LC, Van Marck E, et al. Adamantinoma-like Ewing's sarcoma and Ewing's-like adamantinoma. J Pathol 2001;195(2):218–21.

19. Hazelbag HM, Taminiau AHM, Fleuren GJ, et al. Adamantinoma of the long bones. A clinicopathological study of thirty-two patients with emphasis on histological subtype, precursor lesion, and biological behavior. J Bone Joint Surg Am 1994;76(10):1482–99.

20. Moon NF, Mori H. Adamantinoma of the appendicular skeleton – updated. Clin Orthop Relat Res 1986;204:215–37.

21. Qureshi AA, Shott S, Mallin BA, et al. Current trends in the management of adamantinoma of long bones. J Bone Joint Surg Am 2000;82(8):1122–31.

22. Sarisozen B, Durak K, Ozturk C. Adamantinoma of the tibia in a nine-year-old child. Acta Orthop Belg 2002;68(4):412–6.

23. Kumar D, Mulligan ME, Levine AM, et al. Classic adamantinoma in a 3-year-old. Skeletal Radiol 1998;27(7):406–9.

24. Giardino C. [Cystic adamantinoma of the mandible. Clinical contribution]. Arch Stomatol (Napoli) 1973;14(1–2):43–53 [in Italian].

25. Lavorgna G, Cozzolino A. [A case of recidivous cystic adamantinoma: therapeutic considerations]. Arch Stomatol (Napoli) 1976;17(1–2):55–67 [in Italian].

26. Sica GS, Savastano G, Russo A, et al. [Cystic adamantinoma of the mandible: therapeutic principles]. Arch Stomatol (Napoli) 1983;24(1):19–27 [in Italian].

27. Brain EC, Raymond E, Goldwasser F, et al. [Adamantinoma of the proximal end of the tibia. A case]. Presse Med 1994;23(33):1522–6 [in French].

28. Garces P, Romano CC, Vellet AD, et al. Adamantinoma of the tibia: plain-film, computed tomography and magnetic resonance imaging appearance. Can Assoc Radiol J 1994;45(4):314–7.

29. Judmaier W, Peer S, Krejzi T, et al. MR findings in tibial adamantinoma. A case report. Acta Radiol 1998;39(3):276–8.

30. Campanacci M, Giunti A, Bertoni F, et al. Adamantinoma of the long bones. The experience at the Istituto Ortopedico Rizzoli. Am J Surg Pathol 1981;5(6):533–42.

31. Gebhardt MC, Lord FC, Rosenberg AE, et al. The treatment of adamantinoma of the tibia by wide resection and allograft bone transplantation. J Bone Joint Surg Am 1987;69(8):1177–88.

32. Kanamori M, Antonescu CR, Scott M, et al. Extra copies of chromosomes 7, 8, 12, 19, and 21 are recurrent in adamantinoma. J Mol Diagn 2001;3(1):16–21.

33. Baker PL, Dockerty MB, Coventry MB. Adamantinoma (so-called) of the long bones; review of the literature and report of three new cases. J Bone Joint Surg Am 1954;36(4):704–20.

34. Rock MG, Beabout JW, Unni KK, et al. Adamantinoma. Orthopedics 1983;6:472–7.

35. Makley JT. The use of allografts to reconstruct intercalary defects of long bones. Clin Orthop Relat Res 1985;197:58–75.

36. Gidumal R, Wood MB, Sim FH, et al. Vascularized bone transfer for limb salvage and reconstruction after resection of aggressive bone lesions. J Reconstr Microsurg 1987;3(3):183–8.

37. Goldberg VM, Stevenson S. Natural history of autografts and allografts. Clin Orthop Relat Res 1987;225:7–16.

38. Mnaymneh W, Malinin T. Massive allografts in surgery of bone tumors. Orthop Clin North Am 1989;20(3):455–67.

39. Luzzati A, Mapelli S, Giraldi A. Diaphyseal and metaphyseal hemiresection with autograft reconstruction in the treatment of low grade tumors of the long bones. Ital J Orthop Traumatol 1991;17:81–6.

40. Han CS, Wood MB, Bishop AT, et al. Vascularized bone transfer. J Bone Joint Surg Am 1992;74(10):1441–9.

41. Aldyami E, Abudu A, Grimer RJ, et al. Endoprosthetic replacement of diaphyseal bone defects. Long-term results. Int Orthop 2005;29(1):25–9.
42. Mavrogenis AF, Sakellariou VI, Tsibidakis H, et al. Adamantinoma of the tibia treated with a new intramedullary diaphyseal segmental defect implant. J Int Med Res 2009;37(4):1238–45.
43. Sakellariou VI, Mavrogenis AF, Papagelopoulos PJ. Limb salvage surgery using the intramedullary diaphyseal segmental defect fixation system. J Long Term Eff Med Implants 2008;18(1):59–67.
44. Brigman BE, Horniecek FJ, Gebhardt MC, et al. Allografts about the knee in young patients with high-grade sarcoma. Clin Orthop Relat Res 2004;421:232–9.
45. Erler K, Yildiz C, Baykal B, et al. Reconstruction of defects following bone tumor resections by distraction osteogenesis. Arch Orthop Trauma Surg 2005;125(3): 177–83.
46. Aldlyami E, Abudu A, Grimer RJ, et al. Endoprosthetic replacement of diaphyseal bone defects. Long-term results. Int Orthop 2005;29(1):25–9.
47. Manfrini M, Vanel D, De Paolis M, et al. Imaging of vascularized fibula autograft placed inside a massive allograft in reconstruction of lower limb bone tumors. AJR Am J Roentgenol 2004;182(4):963–70.
48. Donati D, Di Liddo M, Zavatta M, et al. Massive bone allograft reconstruction in high-grade osteosarcoma. Clin Orthop Relat Res 2000;377:186–94.
49. Gebhardt MC, Flugstadt DI, Springfield DS, et al. The use of bone allografts for limb salvage in high-grade extremity osteosarcoma. Clin Orthop Relat Res 1991;270:181–96.
50. Mankin MJ, Gebhardt MC, Jennings LC, et al. Long term results of allograft replacement in the management of bone tumors. Clin Orthop Relat Res 1996; 324:86–97.
51. Thompson RC Jr, Garg A, Clohisy DR, et al. Fractures in large-segment allografts. Clin Orthop Relat Res 2000;370:227–35.
52. San Julian AM, Leyes M, Mora G, et al. Consolidation of massive bone allografts in limb-preserving operations for bone tumours. Int Orthop 1995;19(6):377–82.
53. Ortiz-Cruz E, Gebhardt MC, Jennings LC, et al. The results of transplantation of intercalary allografts after resection of tumors. J Bone Joint Surg Am 1997; 79(1):97–106.
54. Mankin HJ, Doppelt SH, Sullivan TR, et al. Osteoarticular and intercalary allograft transplantation in the management of malignant tumors of bone. Cancer 1982; 50(4):613–30.
55. Hornicek FJ, Gebhardt MC, Tomford WW, et al. Factors affecting nonunion of the allograft-host junction. Clin Orthop Relat Res 2001;382:87–98.
56. Weiss SW, Dorfman HD. Adamantinoma of long bones. An analysis of nine new cases with emphasis on metastasizing lesions and fibrous dysplasia-like changes. Hum Pathol 1977;8(2):141–53.
57. Lokich J. Metastatic adamantinoma of bone to lung? A case report of the natural history and the use of chemotherapy and radiation therapy. Am J Clin Oncol 1994;17(2):157–9.
58. Van Schoor JX, Vallaeys JH, Joos GF, et al. Adamantinoma of the tibia with pulmonary metastases and hypercalcemia. Chest 1991;100(1):279–81.
59. Plump D, Haponik EF, Katz RS, et al. Primary adamantinoma of rib: thoracic manifestations of a rare bone tumor. South Med J 1986;79(3):352–5.

A Simple Adjunct to a Plantar Local Random Flap for Submetatarsal Ulcers

Claire M. Capobianco, DPM[a], Crystal L. Ramanujam, DPM[b],
Thomas Zgonis, DPM, FACFAS[a,b,*]

KEYWORDS

• Foot • Submetatarsal ulcer • Diabetes mellitus • Local flaps
• Diabetic neuropathy

Despite aggressive offloading, diabetic neuropathic plantar ulcerations can be notoriously difficult to resolve permanently. Various plastic surgical techniques are available to accomplish stable, durable, and functional closure of a diabetic foot wound to limit the potential for reulceration, infection, and amputation.[1] When plantar coverage of small soft tissue defects is warranted, the use of a local random flap can be very useful. The authors describe a surgical technique that incorporates the addition of temporary stabilization of the adjacent metatarsophalangeal joint. This technique has been used previously as an adjunct for palmar V-Y advancement flaps in congenital and Dupuytren contractures of the hands.[2]

TECHNIQUE

The patient is positioned supine on the operating table, and a weight-based perioperative antibiotic, typically a first generation cephalosporin, is administered. After initiation of general anesthesia, a nonsterile pneumatic calf tourniquet is applied to the ipsilateral extremity, and the extremity is prepared and draped in a typical sterile manner. After exsanguination of the limb, the tourniquet is inflated to 250 mm Hg. The submetatarsal head ulcer is circumscribed and sharply excised using a full-thickness incision, taking care to avoid skiving of the skin edges. All tissue that appears

---

[a] Division of Podiatric Medicine and Surgery, Department of Orthopaedic Surgery, University of Texas Health Science Center at San Antonio, 7703 Floyd Curl Drive, San Antonio, TX 78229, USA
[b] Division of Podiatric Medicine and Surgery, Department of Orthopaedic Surgery, University of Texas Health Science Center at San Antonio, 7703 Floyd Curl Drive, San Antonio, TX 78229, USA
* Corresponding author. Division of Podiatric Medicine and Surgery, Department of Orthopaedic Surgery, University of Texas Health Science Center at San Antonio, 7703 Floyd Curl Drive, San Antonio, TX 78229.
E-mail address: zgonis@uthscsa.edu (T. Zgonis).

Clin Podiatr Med Surg 27 (2010) 167–172
doi:10.1016/j.cpm.2009.09.004
0891-8422/09/$ – see front matter © 2010 Elsevier Inc. All rights reserved.

necrotic is sharply debrided, and deep soft tissue specimen is sent for Gram staining and aerobic, anaerobic, and fungal cultures. If the metatarsal head is exposed in the base of the ulcer, it is also widely excised and sent for appropriate cultures and histopathologic analysis.

Next, the plantar local random flap is outlined on the skin and a full-thickness incision is performed through the underlying plantar fascia to prevent skin tethering during flap advancement. Perpendicularly oriented septa between the plantar fascia and fat pad are incised to facilitate flap mobility.

The tourniquet is deflated, and meticulous hemostasis is obtained with careful electrocautery and application of topical thrombin. The plantar local random flap is advanced to the defect site using skin hooks and is sutured in place using 2.0 nylon simple interrupted sutures. Forceps are judiciously used during suturing so as not to traumatize the flap.

The ankle is then dorsiflexed to neutral, the toe is stabilized in a plantar-flexed position, and a 0.062 Kirschner wire (K-wire) is retrograded from the distal toe pulp through the phalanges and into the metatarsal head under fluoroscopic guidance. The exposed end of the wire is bent dorsally and covered.

The flap is then dressed with sterile povidone-iodine soaked nonadherent petroleum gauze, multiple fluffed gauzes, and loosely applied gauze roll. A well-padded posterior splint and a plantar cutout to accommodate the plantar-flexed digit are applied. Typically, the patient is discharged and sent home the same day. A strict non–weight-bearing status is maintained for the first 2 weeks in the splint, followed by another 2 weeks in a surgical shoe. Sutures are removed 4 weeks after surgery, and the patient is progressed to flatfoot weight bearing in the surgical shoe. The K-wire is removed in the doctor's office approximately 6 weeks after surgery and when the flap is completely healed (**Fig. 1**).

DISCUSSION

Plantar local random flaps, including well-known V-Y variations, have been well described in the literature, and they play an integral role in soft tissue reconstruction of the diabetic foot. The V-Y local random advancement flap was first described by Atasoy and colleagues[3] in 1970 for reconstruction of fingertip amputations. Since then, the applications of this flap have been further examined and shown to be quite useful in the hand literature.[4–8]

Initially, palmar V-Y advancement flaps were adopted as modifications to the well-known Moberg and Hueston flaps, which were used for digital amputation reconstructions in the late 1960s.[6] This modification allowed for primary closure of the donor site, thus avoiding skin grafting and simplifying the procedure. The use of this flap was also advocated for volar digital pulp avulsions without bone loss,[2,8] postamputation claw nail deformities,[4] thumb tip injuries,[7] proximal volar digital defects,[6] and palmar flexion contractures secondary to congenital causes or Dupuytren disease.[2]

In 1987, Botte and colleagues[4] first described the application of this flap in the foot for reconstruction and closure of a traumatic hallux amputation. The utility of V-Y local advancement flaps for soft tissue defect coverage was further elaborated on for the rearfoot,[9,10] midfoot,[11] forefoot,[12,13] and toes.[3,14,15] Previously, toe fillet and neurovascular island flaps were enlisted for coverage of plantar metatarsal head ulcers. Specifically, Roukis and Zgonis[16] described useful modifications of the traditional great toe fibular flap to allow for reconstruction of infected diabetic plantar forefoot wounds.

The mobility of the V-Y advancement flap must be considered. Although scant literature pertaining to excursion of this flap was published in the foot and ankle literature,

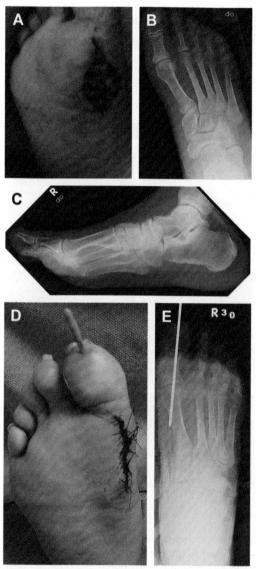

Fig. 1. Clinical appearance (*A*) and preoperative anteroposterior (*B*) and lateral (*C*) radiographic views of the right foot showing the full-thickness ulceration sub–first metatarsal head and after extensive debridement. The first metatarsophalangeal joint was negative for osteomyelitis or septic arthritis as shown by magnetic resonance imaging and bone scintigraphy. Clinical appearance (*D*) and postoperative anteroposterior (*E*) and lateral (*F*) radiographic views showing the plantar O-T local random flap by stabilizing the metatarsophalangeal joint in slight plantarflexion. Clinical appearance (*G*) and postoperative anteroposterior (*H*) and lateral (*I*) radiographic views of the right foot at 1-year follow-up.

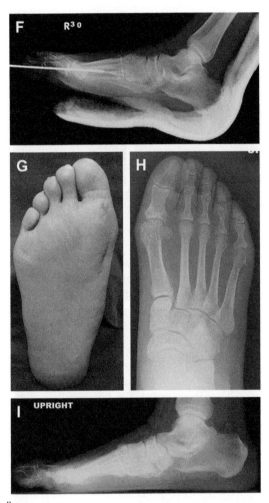

Fig. 1. *(Continued)*

the topic has been addressed more thoroughly in the hand literature. The degree of flap excursion was reported to be from 1.5 to 2.0 cm in the foot[13] and 0.7 to 2.5 cm in the hand, depending on location.[2,4,7] Arguably, the relative thickness of the stratum corneum in the hand, although present, is markedly less than that in the foot, making palmar flaps more supple and potentially prone to easier closure after greater excursion.

A thorough understanding of the arterial anatomy of the plantar skin of the distal forefoot is essential. Much like in the hand, multiple terminal perforating branches of the cutaneous vessels arise deep from the plantar fascia in the foot and travel perpendicularly toward the skin to anastomose with the subdermal plexus. The perforating vessels do not anastomose with the subcutaneous plexus. The perforators are regularly distributed in the distal plantar skin, at approximately 8- to 12-mm increments apart.[13] The vessels are accompanied by corresponding branches of the medial and lateral plantar nerves, which, in a sensate patient, result in a sensate flap.[13] Care must be taken to avoid subcutaneous undermining of the flap, so as not to compromise the perforating blood supply to the skin. The motility gained by the flap ought to be secondary to the transection of the septa anchoring the plantar fascia to the metatarsal heads via the plantar plate. Delicate tissue handling with limited retraction is imperative to prevent tissue necrosis and subsequent flap failure.[15]

Although not explicitly detailed in the operative technique, the first appearance of K-wire temporary stabilization of adjacent joints with V-Y flaps is evident in the images published by Kinoshita and colleagues.[2] The stabilization of the affected or adjacent digit in slight flexion reduces the amount of surface tension across the newly mobilized flap. In doing so, the potential for reactive tension-induced vasospasm is reduced and the flap viability is improved. Because surgeons of the foot and hand are quite familiar with the use of K-wire temporary stabilization for other procedures, using this technique as an adjunct adds a negligible amount of time and effort to the overall surgery. In the foot, the authors recommend stabilizing the adjacent metatarsophalangeal joint in approximately 15° of plantarflexion and removing the fixation in approximately 6 weeks after surgery in a clinical setting under sterile conditions. The joints and adjacent soft tissues must be free of any signs of infection or osteomyelitis before the fixation and must be documented by imaging, intraoperative cultures, and laboratory analysis.

In theory, surgical correction of all the causes contributing to forefoot overload can be an effective method of resolving the recalcitrant plantar ulceration. But in practice, not all patients are reasonable candidates for these significant reconstructive procedures. The role of gastrocnemius or gastrosoleal equinus must be considered in any patient with recalcitrant forefoot ulcerations. When appropriate, gastrocnemius recession can be done in conjunction with the plantar local random flap coverage of the defect and can aid in offloading the forefoot.

In conclusion, the use of local random flaps can provide immediate and durable soft tissue coverage of submetatarsal ulcerations with similar weight bearing plantar skin and minimal donor site morbidity. The addition of a temporary K-wire stabilization of the adjacent metatarsophalangeal joint helps avoid undue tension on the flap during its early phases of incorporation and thus is a valuable adjunctive step in the ultimate success of the flap.

REFERENCES

1. Zgonis T, Stapleton JJ, Roukis TS. Advanced plastic surgery techniques for soft tissue coverage of the diabetic foot. Clin Podiatr Med Surg 2007;24(3):547–68.
2. Kinoshita Y, Kojima T, Matsuura S, et al. Extending the use of the palmar advancement flap with V-Y closure. J Hand Surg Br 1997;22(2):212–8.
3. Atasoy E, Ioakimidis E, Kasdan ML, et al. Reconstruction of the amputated finger tip with a triangular volar flap. A new surgical procedure. J Bone Joint Surg Am 1970;52(52):921–6.
4. Botte MJ, Gellman H. Reconstruction of a traumatic hallux amputation using a plantar V-Y advancement flap. Clin Orthop Relat Res 1987;Jul(220):211–6.
5. Moiemen N, Elliot D. Palmar V-Y reconstruction of proximal defects of the volar aspect of the digits. Br J Plast Surg 1994;47(1):35–41.
6. Bang H, Kojima T, Hayashi H. Palmar advancement flap with V-Y closure for thumb tip injuries. J Hand Surg Am 1992;17(5):933–4.
7. Furlow LT Jr. V-Y "Cup" flap for volar oblique amputation of fingers. J Hand Surg Br 1984;9(3):253–6.
8. Roblin P, Healy CM. Heel reconstruction with a medial plantar V-Y flap. Plast Reconstr Surg 2007;119(3):927–32.

9. Hayashi A, Maruyama Y. Stepladder V-Y advancement flap for repair of postero-plantar heel ulcers. Br J Plast Surg 1997;50(8):657–61.

10. Eroğlu L, Güneren E, Keskin M, et al. The extended V-Y flap for coverage of a mid-plantar defect. Br J Plast Surg 2000;53(8):708–10.

11. Giraldo F, De Haro F, Ferrer A. Opposed transverse extended V-Y plantar flaps for reconstruction of neuropathic metatarsal head ulcers. Plast Reconstr Surg 2001; 108(4):1019–24.

12. Colen LB, Replogle SL, Mathes SJ. The V-Y plantar flap for reconstruction of the forefoot. Plast Reconstr Surg 1988;81(2):220–8.

13. Bharathi RR, Jerome JT, Kalson NS, et al. V-Y advancement flap coverage of toe-tip injuries. J Foot Ankle Surg 2009;48(3):368–71.

14. Botte MJ, Gellman H. Reconstruction of a traumatic hallux amputation using a plantar V-Y advancement flap. Clin Orthop Relat Res 1987;220:211–6.

15. Zgonis T, Stapleton JJ, Rodriguez RH, et al. Plastic surgery reconstruction of the diabetic foot. AORN J 2008;87(5):951–66.

16. Roukis TS, Zgonis T. Modifications of the great toe fibular flap for diabetic forefoot and toe reconstruction. Ostomy Wound Manage 2005;51(6):30–2.

Index

Clin Podiatr Med Surg 27 (2010) 173–181
doi:10.1016/S0891-8422(09)00113-X
0891-8422/09/$ – see front matter © 2010 Elsevier Inc. All rights reserved.

podiatric.theclinics.com

Printed and bound by CPI Group (UK) Ltd, Croydon, CR0 4YY
03/10/2024
01040463-0015

D

Diabetes mellitus, submetatarsal ulcers in, plantar local flap for, **167–172**
Dobbs approach, for congenital vertical talus, 81–82, 152–154
Duchenne's muscular dystrophy, equinus deformity in, 29

E

Equinus deformity, **25–42**
  biomechanical examination in, 46
  causes of, 25–26
  in arthrogryposis, 31
  in cerebral palsy, 29–30
  in Charcot-Marie-Tooth disease, 29
  in clubfoot, 31
  in fibular hemimelia, 32–33
  in flatfoot, 30–31
  in flexible flatfoot, 13–14, 61–64
  in muscular dystrophy, 29
  in spinal bifida, 30
  in tarsal coalitions, 113
  osseous, 31
  physical examination in, 26–27
  radiography for, 28
  spastic, 29–30
  toe walking with, 28–29
  treatment of
    complications of, 39–40
    conservative, 33–36
    external fixation in, 40–41
    surgical, 36–40, 61–64
  versus equinus contracture, 26
  versus pseudoequinus deformity, 31
Evans calcaneal osteotomy
  for flexible flatfoot, 68–70
  for skewfoot deformity, 99–100, 102
Exercise, for flexible flatfoot, 60
External fixation, for equinus deformity, 40–41

F

Femur, biomechanics of, in flexible flatfoot, 53
Fibular hemimelia, equinus deformity with, 32–33
Flatfoot deformity. *See* Pediatric pes planovalgus deformity.
Flexible flatfoot
  acquired
    clinical features of, 47–48
    diagnosis of, 51–52
    in trauma, 54
  asymptomatic, 8–9
  biomechanics of, 52–54

Moving?

Make sure your subscription moves with you!

To notify us of your new address, find your **Clinics Account Number** (located on your mailing label above your name), and contact customer service at:

Email: journalscustomerservice-usa@elsevier.com

800-654-2452 (subscribers in the U.S. & Canada)
314-447-8871 (subscribers outside of the U.S. & Canada)

Fax number: 314-447-8029

Elsevier Health Sciences Division
Subscription Customer Service
3251 Riverport Lane
Maryland Heights, MO 63043